THE
GROUNDING
COMPANION

QUARTO.COM

© 2025 Quarto Publishing Group USA Inc.
Text © 2025 Donna Raskin
Illustration © 2025 Beatrice Müller

First published in 2025 by Fair Winds Press, an imprint of The Quarto Group,
100 Cummings Center, Suite 265-D, Beverly, MA 01915, USA.
T (978) 282-9590 F (978) 283-2742

Fair Winds Press titles are also available at discount for retail, wholesale,
promotional, and bulk purchase. For details, contact the Special Sales Manager by
email at specialsales@quarto.com or by mail at The Quarto Group, Attn: Special
Sales Manager, 100 Cummings Center, Suite 265-D, Beverly, MA 01915, USA.

29 28 27 26 25   1 2 3 4 5

ISBN: 978-0-7603-9310-9

Digital edition published in 2025
eISBN: 978-0-7603-9311-6

Library of Congress Control Number: 2024944955

Cover Design: Samantha J Bednarek
Illustration: Bea Müller @ soleyandthebear

Printed in Malaysia

The information in this book is for educational purposes only. It is not intended
to replace the advice of a physician or medical practitioner. Please see your
health-care provider before beginning any new health program.

THE
GROUNDING
COMPANION

Tap Into the Healing Power of Nature for Health, Longevity, and Vitality

DONNA RASKIN

Illustrated by
Bea Müller

FAIR WINDS

CONTENTS

Chapter 4

Grounding Locations 056

Chapter 5

Grounding Foods 112

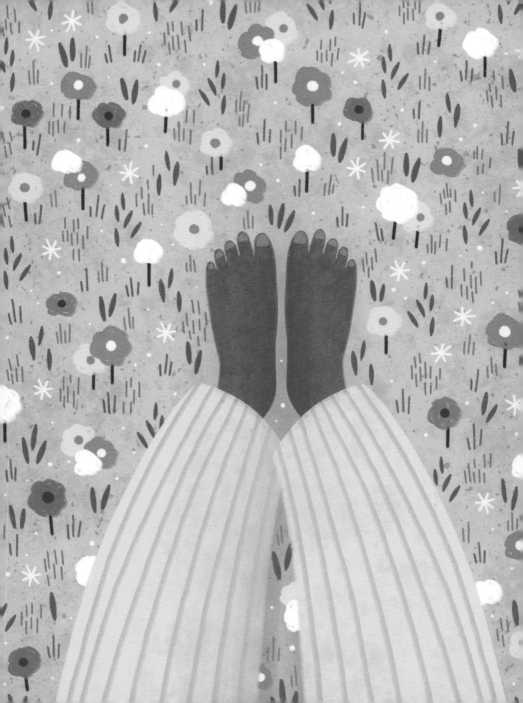

INTRODUCTION

---

*"Find your place on the planet. Dig in,
and take responsibility from there."*

GARY SNYDER

Before you read all the science about grounding and the ailments it can improve, here's a quick experiment to do so you can fully experience the reality of what it feels like to ground yourself. In a perfect world, yes, you would do this outside, but it's okay for this example to just be a few "good enough" moments. First, take off your shoes and socks. Then, sit down and put your feet flat on the floor, even if that means you are sitting mostly off the chair or couch. Relax your shoulders and take a few deep breaths. Although you probably felt fine a minute ago, pay attention to how it feels to sit with your feet in contact with the floor. Are you calmer? Do you feel more centered? Most importantly, now that your feet are solidly in contact with the floor, are you more aware of where you are? This is what Ram Dass, the former Harvard University professor and spiritual writer, meant when he said, "Be here now."

He meant that you will gain happiness, inner peace, and better health when you let go of the distraction of phones and screens and instead connect your body to your place on earth. Of course, grounding is not a miracle cure, but it is a practice that can improve chronic illnesses such as inflammation and anxiety and immediate problems such as jet lag.

Grounding is like being lost and then suddenly realizing exactly where you are. You are here. In one spot on earth. That awareness can bring you peace and serenity, as if your energy and the energy around you were swirling and suddenly settles like a blanket around your shoulders, all because you placed your feet gently on the ground and connected to the energy of the earth.

Although there is a specific scientific meaning to grounding—and we will explain the detailed research in this book—we will also open the umbrella to include other ways people connect to earth. Specifically, though, some grounding research has found that when the human body is in contact with earth's natural electric charge, it stabilizes the circulation of human energy in the body, which may reduce inflammation, alleviate pain, and improve general wellness.

Now, having said that, all the methods we grouped under grounding, which is sometimes called earthing, have scientific validity. Research has shown that routinely walking barefoot outdoors, using inexpensive grounding systems indoors while sleeping or sitting, forest bathing, water bathing, and swimming can reduce symptoms of many illnesses.

Of course, that doesn't mean scientists or medical doctors have been able to find out why these cures work. Some of the solutions are anecdotal. If you just "feel better" when you are outside, a double-blind, university-funded research experiment may not be able to measure just how differently you feel (especially in comparison to how you would have felt by not going outside), nor will a scientist necessarily be able to explain exactly why you improved.

Although there are clear studies demonstrating that connecting with the natural earth can improve your health, science is still learning the exact details about electromagnetism and its effects, both positive and negative, on the human body.

Does that matter? It depends. Some of us believe our own experience while others require nonbiased proof. Right now, there is a lot of scientific evidence about most of these practices, and where there is science, you will find the research in this book.

Whichever type of person you are, you will find plenty of ideas about how to ground yourself when you need to relieve anxiety, make better food choices for your overall health, and travel around the world to places that have provided respite to millions of people.

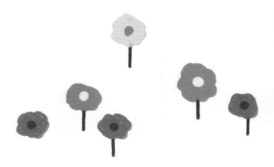

1

THE SCIENCE BEHIND GROUNDING

—

"I sing the body electric."
WALT WHITMAN

Although the term *grounding* refers specifically to the connection between your body and the earth through electromagnetic energy, in this book we are going to explore all the ways in which your body interacts with and is healed by a variety of landscapes and elements, including water, air, and earth. But first, you should understand the specific and detailed meaning of grounding, that is, the ways in which being in electromagnetic connection with the earth may benefit your health.

According to the World Health Organization (WHO), invisible electromagnetic fields are all around us; they occur when waves of electric and magnetic energy move together. These energy fields surround us all the time. It is the earth's magnetic field that makes a compass work, and animals use electromagnetism to know where they should fly and where they should swim.

When you walk through rain, you get wet. When you walk through a hard wind, your body is blown back. You can see and feel rain, just like you can feel wind and see its effect on nearby trees, branches, and leaves. Although you can't see electricity (unless there is lightning in the sky) and you may not necessarily feel its effect, that doesn't mean it's not interacting with you! In fact, your body is engaged with electromagnetism all the time.

This is partly why it has been difficult for scientists to fully understand the potential effects of electromagnetism on themselves and others. In fact, for generations, electricity, magnetic fields, and electromagnetic fields only occurred naturally. Today, though, people are exposed to all sorts of artificial sources of electromagnetic fields, from small cell phones to large power grids. As WHO writes on its website, "Everyone is exposed to a complex mix of weak electric and magnetic fields, both at home and at work, from the generation and transmission of electricity . . . (in) domestic appliances and industrial equipment, to telecommunications and broadcasting."

Do all of those fields, both weak and strong, affect your health, including your emotional health? Yes, they do. Very strong electromagnetic fields have proven to be dangerous to humans, animals, and plants. Also, these fields have radiation, which is the emission of energy as waves or subatomic particles. There are two general kinds of electromagnetic radiation: ionizing and nonionizing. Ionizing radiation can knock electrons out of their orbit around an atom. This can be damaging to a body's cells. Nonionizing radiation has enough energy to move atoms in a molecule around and cause them to vibrate, which makes the atom heat up, but not enough to remove the electrons from the atoms.

So, if these electromagnetic fields and their radiation can alter the alignment of atoms, can they affect your cells? Of course. For example, the Environmental Protection Agency (EPA) reports that extremely low frequency electromagnetic fields are possibly carcinogenic because they are associated with higher rates of childhood leukemia. How do scientists know this? Again, because not all electricity is man-made. If you were hit by lightning, your body would respond to the shock of electricity by having a range of injuries, including hearing loss, cardiac arrest, and behavioral changes. That's because we have an electrical system in our bodies, and like all things human, it's a delicate balance of energy that keeps us healthy.

THE HEART AND ELECTRICITY

The human body is a repository of electricity. Nerves transmit electrical impulses, and most bodily functions require the movement of charged particles. It's not only the brain that runs on electricity; so does the heart, which is exactly why a stopped heart is brought back to life by a defibrillator, a machine that applies an electrical current to the heart. It's also why, if you have a pacemaker, you shouldn't stand near a microwave—when a pacemaker is exposed to high levels of energy, it can malfunction.

To remain healthy, the human body has a network of cells called the cardiac conduction system, which is the heart's electrical system. Cells in this system generate electrical impulses, sending signals through the heart to pump blood at specific speeds. Your heartbeat is entirely dependent on your body's electrical system. This system is part of the autonomic nervous system, which is unconscious and affects not only your heart, but also your breathing and digestion. This is partly why, when you feel anxious, you may start to breathe more shallowly or get an upset stomach.

Just as your heart relies on electricity to pump properly, the neurons in your brain use electrical charges and ions to work properly. Because electricity is partly responsible for your brain's health and function, over the years, doctors and scientists have turned to electrical stimulation to improve (or harm) the brain's function. Brain stimulation can improve mood disorders, such as depression and schizophrenia, among other issues.

Cells, which are made up of atoms, are, of course, what makes up our entire body, from heart to brain and everything in between. Some of those cells are naturally healthy, while others contain free radicals. Scientists now know that free radicals are responsible for a host of health issues, and they have long known that cells are "electric." Scientists used to believe that only nerve cells in the brain and muscle cells, such as the heart, were electric, but now it's clear that every cell has one part that works like a little battery. In fact, our bodies are electric just like the earth and its atmosphere. When you slide your feet on a rug, touch someone else, and get a "shock," then you and your friend have become electrical conductors.

WHAT HAPPENS WHEN CELLS GET SICK?

If healthy cells include a little electric charge, what happens to the electricity in unhealthy cells? Well, the answer might have something to do with free radicals, although this type of research is truly in its infancy.

Free radicals are cellular waste molecules that have an unpaired electron. Their positive charge needs to be neutralized by another electron. To fight free radicals, you need antioxidants. You can get antioxidants through food, but you can also get them by grounding to the earth, which has a continuous supply of negatively charged

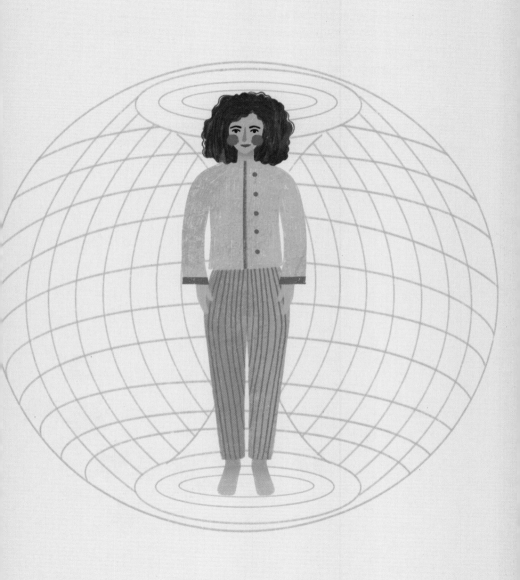

ions and electrons. When free radicals overwhelm a physical system, typically an organ such as the skin, heart, or kidneys, that system begins to suffer from oxidative stress. In fact, free radicals can alter all parts of the human body, down to your DNA, and trigger several diseases.

Preliminary research has found that electromagnetic fields can cause free radicals and oxidative stress in the body. Again, this type of research is just beginning, but it is one of the reasons some scientists believe grounding—having a healthy connection to the earth's electrical field—can be helpful to people's health.

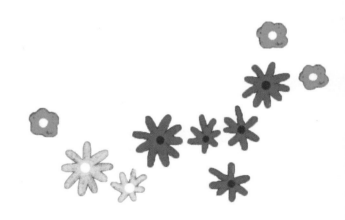

AN ABBREVIATED HISTORY OF GROUNDING

Technically, grounding is a therapy in which the human body connects, through electromagnetism, to the ground or a grounding mat. Some medical historians date it back to the Chinese concept of *qi*, or vital energy. Others believe that what we think of as "grounding" or "earthing" dates back to the 1990s, when a cable TV salesman named Clint Ober began to consider how his experience in grounding cables might help improve people's health.

Although Ober has written about his research with doctors and other doctors have done studies about grounding and earthing, there is, as mentioned, a dearth of double-blind confirmed studies about the effects of grounding. Still, over the last few years, more academics have published research about grounding and earthing in respected journals, including *Biomedical Journal* and *Journal of Inflammation Research*. For example, doctors Gaétan Chevalier, Gregory Melvin, and Tiffany Barsotti published a randomized, double-blind pilot study in *Health* in 2023 showing that one-hour contact with the earth's surface improves inflammation and blood flow.

You can expect that the research about the positive effects of grounding will explode over the next decade. Following are all the very many ways grounding and grounding practices will likely improve your health.

2

SIMPLE GROUNDING TECHNIQUES

"Creativity is seeing what everyone else has seen and thinking what no one else has thought."

ALBERT EINSTEIN

There are numerous ways to ground yourself, and this chapter will explore many easy and accessible ones. In its broadest sense, grounding yourself doesn't have to mean literally standing on the ground. You can simply touch something from nature, such as a smooth stone or a small branch. Grounding yourself is especially wonderful when you can be in a natural setting, but there are plenty of methods to use when you can't be outside.

How you ground yourself and whether you do it as a regular daily practice or on an as-needed basis is up to you, of course. Some grounding techniques, such as meditation and gardening, are wonderful daily habits, while others, like putting your feet on the floor and noticing items around you, are best in specific situations. You can't, for example, garden when you're in your office and have an anxiety attack. On the other hand, you can have a plant or two on your desk so that you are reminded of grounding techniques while you're at work.

The point is to have a variety of grounding techniques that feel personal and useful to you so that when you feel anxious or upset, you can take a few minutes to connect with yourself and the earth.

PUTTING YOUR FEET ON THE FLOOR

At its essence, grounding is putting your body in contact with the earth. That could be lying down, standing, or simply sitting in a chair and putting your feet on the floor. You, like many others, may spend very little time with your feet actually on the ground. For example, you sleep on a bed, you drive in a car, and it's possible you sit on a couch or at a desk where your feet are either reclining with you or don't touch the floor. Even though the floor is not as grounded as the actual earth, you can still ground yourself by putting your feet on the floor.

Here are some ways to make sure you get more conscious contact with the floor.

IN THE MORNING: When you wake up, put both feet on the floor by your bed and, before actually taking a step, stay on the edge of the bed for a minute or two. Take a few deep breaths and feel contact so that you give yourself time before your day begins to not only connect with the earth beneath you, but also with yourself.

TO IMPROVE THIS GROUNDING EXPERIENCE, TRY TOE/HEEL BREATHING:

1. Take a slow inhale, and, while you do that, lift your toes away from the floor. You should feel the inhale in your belly and chest; they should expand.

2. On an exhale, lower your toes slowly. Feel yourself get smaller without the breath to puff you up. Do this five times.

3. Then, on an inhale, lift your heels. On an exhale, lower your heels.

4. Finally, take another slow five breaths with your feet fully on the floor.

It is likely you will feel more centered and able to start your day with less worry.

DURING THE DAY: Whether you are home with children or at a job (or doing any of the million other things a person can do during the day), there are always moments that can upset, distract, or worry you. Understanding ways to ground yourself when this happens is a helpful coping tool.

First, consider carrying a stone or small stick to hold when you need to ground yourself. Although lots of people use fidgets, choosing an object from nature is far more helpful. This is an especially good exercise if you are at a desk or somewhere it isn't easy to take a walk.

TO TAKE A QUIET WALK WITHOUT LEAVING YOUR SEAT:

1. Sit on a chair with your feet on the floor. Press one foot slowly into the ground while you lift the other foot and lower leg up.

2. Release the first foot and press the other foot on the floor. Try to initiate movement from your upper legs and hips. While you're doing this, inhale and exhale.

3. It is up to you how fast or slow you do these motions. Do this as long as you feel comfortable.

AT NIGHT: Many people have trouble falling asleep and dissolving into dreamland.

You can lie on the floor of your bedroom, but this grounding activity is specifically for lying on your bed before you go to sleep. This way, you won't have to move and you can simply drift off.

In this meditation, you will ground by surrounding yourself with pillows, so make sure you have a variety of pillows to use. They don't even have to be bed pillows; maybe you have small pillows on your couch, for example. These are the places and pillows you will need:

- Under your neck and head—supportive and soft
- Under your knees—supportive, pretty high
- Under your arms and hands—the same height and density on both sides
- Under your ankles—very soft, not too high; your feet should rest on it, too
- Side sleeper? Consider putting a pillow between your knees, and keep one under your neck and feet.

Place the pillows on your bed, under your covers, and then arrange yourself with the pillows in their correct spots. Once you're settled, you should feel like you're being supported and like you don't have to hold your own weight. This will definitely take some time to get right. Don't rush, and if you find something doesn't work, then adjust.

WHEN YOU'RE READY, BEGIN THE MEDITATION:

1. Inhale through your nose slowly and exhale through your mouth slowly. On the inhale, try to

imagine that your breath is going all the way to your toes and fingers. When you exhale, you should sink into the pillows.

2. As you relax, imagine that you are outdoors with a world of stars above you. Visualize the moon protecting you. You are grounded to the earth and to the sky.

WALKING BAREFOOT

Taking a walk almost always feels good, and grounding research has found that taking a barefoot walk feels even better. Make no mistake, shoes are great. They protect our feet from rough ground and, in many cases, can help our gait by adding support and bounce. Nevertheless, our feet—and our bodies—love the bare earth. Whether it's on grass or sand, our feet are happiest when they touch the ground.

In fact, a 2019 study published in *Landscape Research* explains that although most academic studies that explore nature and feelings of restoration focus primarily on the visual and sound experience, the importance of touch should not be overlooked. People who stood barefoot on the ground reported higher levels of connection and restoration.

Typically, when we think of touch, we consider the importance of skin-to-skin touch, which has been shown to help babies bond with their parents. Extensive research has found that touch lowers heart rate and blood pressure. We feel calmer when we are physically connected to other humans (in a safe and consensual manner, of course). Our immune systems are strengthened by positive touch. Touching those we love signals that we are physically one.

We also gain a sense of connectedness and calm when we touch the earth. Standing barefoot on the ground, which can include sand, dirt, or grass, transmits an electromagnetic connection beneficial to our bodies. According to a 2018 study published in *Complementary Therapies in Medicine*, standing on the beach with wet feet reduced the body's electrical resistance by 94 percent. It's possible, although more research needs to be done, that we feel better with our feet in the sand and on the ground because of our body's electromagnetic response.

TRY THIS SILENT WALKING MEDITATION, WHICH YOU CAN DO BAREFOOT OR IN SHOES:

1. Try to walk slowly. As you walk, be sure to keep your shoulders down away from your ears, so that your neck isn't crunched. Gently engage your abdominals and make sure your rear end isn't tilted out, but is tucked toward your hips. This motion should then encourage you to lift your chest.

2. While you walk, especially if you're barefoot, vary your attention between feeling the ground beneath your feet and the weight of your body as you step down. Of course, you'll have to look up and pay attention to your surroundings, but while you do that, also take the time to be aware of the ground and your steps.

3. If you find that you are too conscious of what's around you rather than your steps, consider following a repetitive path, such as going up and down your street or walking in a wide circle in a park. Walking in a pattern, such as a labyrinth, is a tradition in many cultures. You can find labyrinths in some churches and gardens.

SLEEPING
ON THE GROUND

If you love to go camping, it's likely you are comfortable sleeping on the ground. One thing you might consider is traveling to a Night Sky Park where you will see more stars than you would in other locations. Is it possible to be grounded when you're looking at the sky? Of course it is. In some ways, it will make you even more aware of being grounded on earth because you will be looking at proof that you are on planet Earth.

Looking at the stars is also an easy way to experience awe, and according to research, awe is good for your health. In the book *Awe: The New Science of Everyday Wonder and How It Can Transform Your Life*, psychologist Dacher Keltner explains how awe calms our nervous system and releases oxytocin. This is the hormone that floods through a new mother when she breastfeeds. It is the hormone that bonds us when we fall in love. Keltner also found that when we experience awe, we begin to breathe more deeply and our heart rate slows.

Sometimes awe happens unexpectedly, but more frequently, we have to search for it. And one guarantee of awe is looking up at the night sky to acknowledge the vast universe in which we are grounded to earth.

Another benefit of awe? It gives us a push in the direction away from our own ego. When we look at the sky, we are forced to recognize that the world exists outside of our own perception of our life's importance. The world is going to go on without you, which is often a scary thought. At first. Continue to meditate on this idea. It frees you to value what you have or recognize that you can make changes. You can be whoever you want to be under the stars.

If you don't like camping or aren't able to, you can try sleeping on the floor of your house sometimes. According to the Sleep Foundation, some research has shown a firm sleep surface, such as a

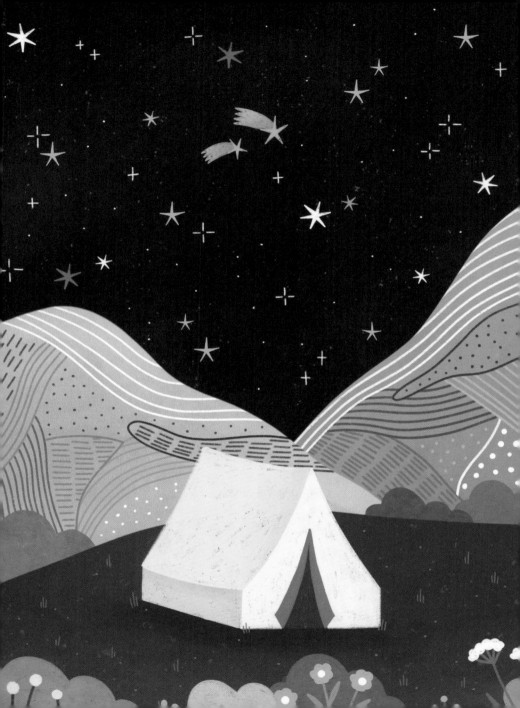

floor, may be beneficial to your back. This is especially true if your mattress is very soft and old and likely not firm enough to support your body weight. Sleeping on the ground or the floor is also beneficial if it's very hot out. The ground is cooler, and, of course, heat rises.

USING A
GROUNDING MAT

The surface of the earth has a negative electric charge, and grounding mats have the same, so a grounding mat brings the experience of walking barefoot outside into your home or office. Putting your bare feet on the mat connects you to it electrically, which is similar to putting your feet on the ground. The connection means electrons flow from the mat to your body.

Grounding mats usually have a rubber backing. The rest of the mat conducts electricity to your feet through a grounding wire that you plug into an outlet. Some mats come with special adapters to ensure that the electricity is properly grounded. There are also other sizes, including wristbands, yoga mats, and mats that are big enough to sleep on.

But is standing on a mat as beneficial as standing on a forest floor or on sand or in lake water? Well, yes and no. Even most grounding mat manufacturers would likely say that a mat is not the same as being in the woods. That's because the benefits of being in nature are exponential. It's not just putting your feet on the earth. It's also the exposure to trees, fresh air, and the movement of wind, among other elements. However, if you can't get outside or if you suspect that regularly grounding yourself will reduce high levels of inflammation, then mats are a great option.

If you do try a grounding mat, consider using it with a meditation rather than just a surface under your feet while you work or do the dishes. Invite all the benefits of grounding into your life, just as you would when you go outside and walk.

SWIMMING

Many people love to swim, and swimming, whether it's merely lounging in water or doing a vigorous butterfly stroke, has proven benefits. According to the American College of Sports Medicine, swimming can improve cardiovascular fitness, increase muscular strength and endurance, and, depending on your skill, burn a significant number of calories. Because it is low impact (there is resistance from the water, but you are weightless), swimming is a terrific way to stay fit, often if you need to rehab from an injury.

Research shows that swimming also helps relieve stress and eases arthritis, and it is a wonderful way for older people, who might suffer from balance issues or be unable to lift their own body weight, to get resistance exercise, such as strength training. Additionally, a 2023 study published in *Physical Sciences* found that rats with severe tissue damage from electromagnetic radiation had reduced signs of oxidative stress and liver cell damage after swimming.

Of course, swimming in non-chemically treated water, whether a lake or an ocean, is healthier than swimming in water with chlorine. But this only holds true when the water you swim in is healthy itself, not polluted. Still, even the fittest people benefit from pool workouts.

Does swimming have any grounding benefits? Clearly, if you swim in a lake or the ocean, you can feel an emotional and physical connection to nature, and there is extensive data backing up those benefits to health. It seems that being in water modulates the oxidative stress brought on by swimming. In other words, exercising in water is less stressful on your body than exercising on land. That may be because of the lack of impact, but it may also be due to some of the ways in which our bodies respond to water itself.

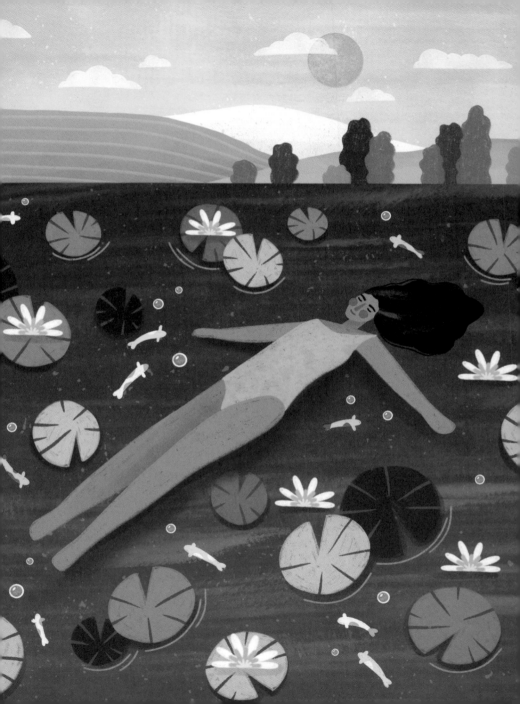

The human body gets most of its resistance to electricity through the skin, but being in water changes that completely. In fact, being in water makes you much more sensitive to electricity, which is why you have to get out of a body of water if there is lightning. Salt water conducts more electricity than fresh water or pool water, so you are safer in the ocean than in other bodies of water.

Therefore, the idea of being "grounded" in the most conservative use of the term in water is impossible. But because swimming has also been shown to reduce symptoms of anxiety and depression, you can consider it a general grounding experience. In fact, because pools must be both grounded and bonded to reduce the likelihood of electric shock, you may benefit from that type of swimming as much as you would by swimming in a natural body of water.

Nevertheless, recently some proponents of "structured" water have begun to tout its benefits. Their argument is that this water, which has been magnetized, exposed to infrared or ultraviolet light, stored in gemstone water bottles, or simply exposed to sunlight, is as close to unpolluted as possible. According to a 2021 paper published in *The Journal of Animal Science*, magnetized water doesn't stay magnetized for long and although it does appear to have positive benefits on the endurance of various animals, no one knows how this translates to people. Also, the magnification required to reach the levels that were tested are out of the reach of most individuals. There is no reliable, double-blind study about this type of water. In fact, is it even water? The chemical formula for water is H_2O, but the formula for structured water, according to advertisements, is H_3O_2. Therefore, "structured" water is not essentially water.

Of course, being in and drinking water is important—we are water. Drinking filtered water is best. Also, be aware that drinking water that has been left in a water bottle in a hot car is definitely not safe, according to the National Institutes of Health.

BATHING

Although it's similar to swimming, bathing is, in fact, different in one specific way: You don't exercise in a bath. Instead, the benefits are specifically about being immersed in water. There are multiple types of baths—cold, hot, thermal, salt—and they are all good for you.

Researchers have found that regular exposure to cold baths helps stimulate the antioxidant barrier and produces positive adaptive changes to the antioxidant capacity of winter swimmers. According to a 2022 literature review study published in the *International Journal of Circumpolar Health*, cold water immersion can positively affect the reduction and/or transformation of body fat, which may be protective against diabetes and heart disease. Taking cold baths positively affects the immune system, as it builds tolerance against stress and respiratory infections.

Likewise, according to a 2020 study published in *Heart*, Japanese people who regularly took baths had considerably lower risks of both heart disease and stroke. According to the Cleveland Clinics, baths are beneficial for a few reasons. First, by ridding your body of dead skin cells, you are also removing skin irritation and inflammation. Also, a warm bath actually helps you sleep by pulling the heat from the core of your body, which lowers your temperature, leading to better sleep.

Bathing, however, should not be an everyday habit, nor should you stay in the water too long, according to the research. Soaking in water for too long or too frequently can dry out your skin.

If you enjoy taking baths, consider it a grounding ritual. You might want to pair it with other grounding practices, such as meditation, to further improve its benefits.

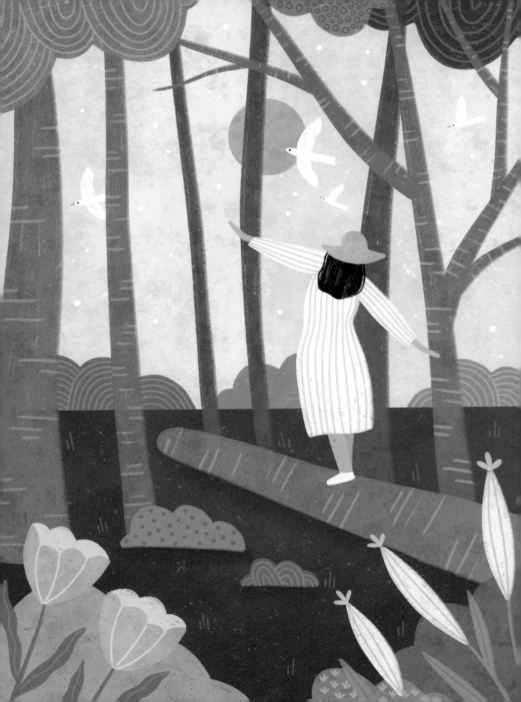

FOREST BATHING

If you've ever taken a walk and found yourself surrounded by nature with no artificial light source or man-made noise, then you know how meaningful an experience it is to be bathed in nature. In this case, of course, *bathe* refers to immersion.

Most of the time, we are in cities, which are almost entirely man-made, or we are in suburbs and the country, which are a combination. A farm, for example, may have a lot of land, but it has been affected by the work of people, with buildings and a landscape filled with crops. Even animals on a farm are not typically in their natural habitat.

Forest bathing means spending time in an all-natural atmosphere that fully surrounds you. A medically proven practice that improves both mental and physical health, forest bathing requires that you unplug from technology and use your senses to experience the natural world. According to a 2017 study, people who spend time in nature report feeling more energetic, having better overall health, and, perhaps most significantly, having a more meaningful sense of purpose.

Despite the promise of technology to "connect" us, technology has taken away from what truly connects us: nature. When we are in nature, we feel connected to not only the world but also to others and ourselves. We can be "addicted" to cell phones and other screens, but we can't become "addicted" to nature—there is no downside to being outside.

This may seem ironic because most outside settings are filled with stimulation—trees, the sounds of birds, different walking surfaces—but it's actually modern urban and office environments that give us sensory overload. The fluorescent lights, the noise, and the lack of nature itself lead to feelings of tension. According to a study in *Frontiers of Psychology*, we actually focus and concentrate better in nature.

As mentioned, *grounding* refers to having your feet on the ground so that the electrical energy of the earth can interact with the electrical system of your body, but even if you wear shoes when you're outside, you can still forest bathe. In fact, you can do this even if you aren't in a forest. All you need to do is notice the nature around you, because, again, the idea of forest bathing is about connecting with the world using your senses. You will need to take a walk somewhere with natural light, some trees, and, if possible, ground rather than pavement under your feet. Then, focus on touching some of the plant leaves and bark; smelling the scent of the earth and flowers; listening to birds, other animals, and the movement of the plants in the breeze; and looking closely at the world around you.

If you live somewhere without a park or a lot of green space, studies have shown that even looking at images of nature can help calm anxiety. Consider cutting pictures of nature out of magazines or meditating while looking at screen savers of nature. There are many meditation videos on YouTube that make use of both the sounds and scenes of natural habitats. You can add to that experience by listening to sounds of nature while looking at it too.

GARDENING

There are few healthier activities than gardening: putting your hands in the dirt, listening to the outside world, planting flowers and vegetables that support the birds, and growing your own food. It is truly a connection to earth.

Numerous studies have shown that people who garden are happier and live longer, healthier lives than those who don't. For example, a 2022 study published in *Preventive Medicine Reports* found that gardening has psychotherapeutic benefits, improves mental health, and enhances psychological well-being, and that this is true for participants of all ages.

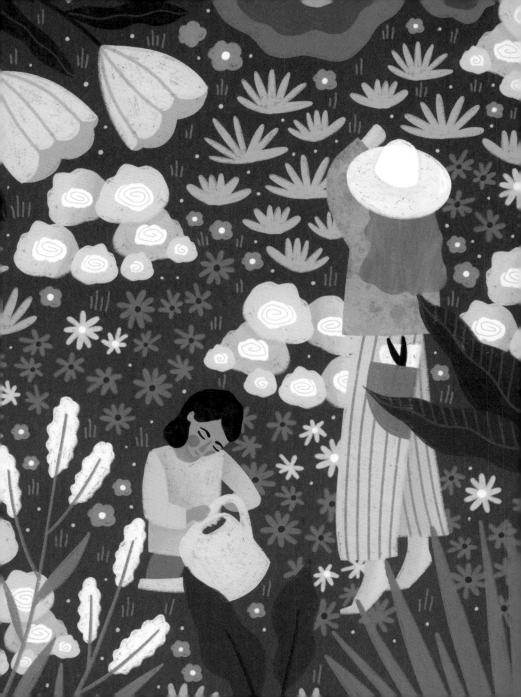

Fortunately, even if you live in a city, you can garden. Indoor plants and container gardens on patios and windowsills can bring just as much happiness as a larger outdoor garden. There are also community gardens in many cities, and this means getting not only the physical benefits of gardening but also the social and emotional benefits of connecting with your neighbors.

Gardening is, typically, a low-intensity type of exercise, although, of course, if you plant large bushes and small trees you can push the intensity up. If you plant a vegetable garden, you will have healthy food to eat.

Finally, one of the most beneficial aspects of gardening is connecting to the rhythms of the days and the seasons. Gardening requires attention to the land and the plants, and you have to know when plants, whether flower or vegetable, will best succeed. Gardening is a grounding technique that bring a few minutes to a few hours of connecting to the earth every day. You are, quite literally, grounding yourself.

YOGA

Like other forms of exercise, yoga improves heart health, balance, and flexibility. It has also been shown to improve numerous health conditions, such as cardiovascular issues, arthritis, and back pain, which often stand in the way of people getting other types of exercise.

Yoga is also deeply relaxing, as it is considered a mind-body practice. That is, you are connecting your breath to your movement so that you consciously lower your stress while holding a pose or transitioning from one pose to another.

The word *yoga*, from ancient Sanskrit, is often translated as "yoke" or "union," which may refer to bringing together the breath with movement, or it may imply the connection of the yogi to the uni-

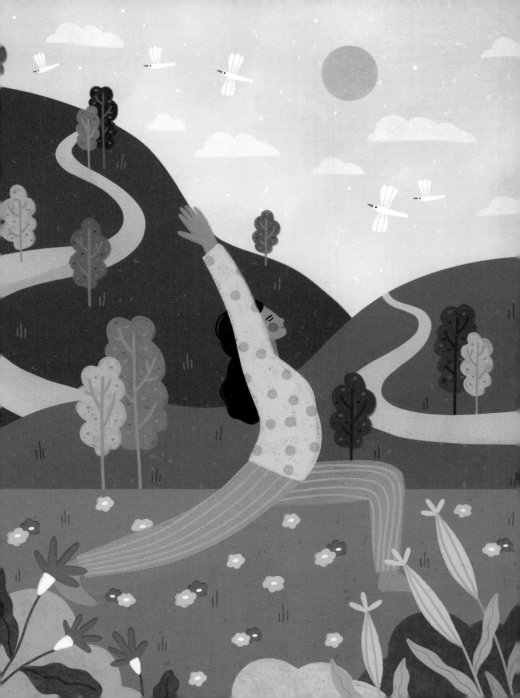

verse. Regardless of the word's meaning, yoga grounds you to earth and to the present moment.

Yoga brings you into a balanced, centered state that includes a connection to yourself and to the wider world—the om. *Om* is considered the sound of creation, the sound of the universe and the earth. Like grounding, which is an energy, om is a frequency and a vibration. From om comes all other vibrations. Remember, when yoga was first created, there was no understanding of "electricity." Being grounded would not have had a meaning that connected to the scientific properties of the earth. But yoga was first designed as a grounding exercise to help adherents release any energy so that they could get ready to sit in meditation.

MEDITATION

Just as there are many forms of yoga, there are also many forms of meditation. They are all designed to help you either focus or empty your mind to bring about relaxation and better health. Meditation is not religious, although some religions incorporate meditation practices into their customs.

Meditation is thousands of years old, but over the last half century, medical research has proven that people who meditate have better cardiovascular and brain health. It has been shown to help with post-traumatic stress disorder and anxiety. In fact, brain scans of people who meditate show that they have greater neural connections than those who don't.

Grounding is a type of meditation because putting your feet on the earth and connecting with nature benefits your state of mind in much the way meditation does. In fact, many grounding practices include meditation. Just like meditation, grounding refers to the ability to be present in the now without distraction.

SOME FORMS OF MEDITATION INCLUDE:

- **MINDFULNESS**—Practicing mindfulness meditation means sitting with your eyes open and trying to let go of your thoughts. To do this, you'll notice something, let's say the pattern of the floor, and you'll simply let that thought go rather than holding on to it. You are trying to "empty" your mind. The "mindfulness" aspect refers to paying attention to the world around you but not grasping onto any one thing or idea.

- **GUIDED**—During a guided meditation, a teacher (or recorded voice) will ask you to listen to and follow their words. This also takes you out of your own mind and into a state of relaxation. Some guided meditations include body scans, white light, and imagining nature or a road. This can sometimes be easier for people who are new to meditation to master because they don't have to "empty" their minds.

- **TRANSCENDENTAL**—Transcendental Meditation, or TM, is a form of silent meditation developed in the 1950s by Maharishi Mahesh Yogi, who later became famous as the yogi to the Beatles, David Lynch, and Howard Stern, among others. When you practice, you simply sit and repeat a word (mantra) to yourself. That phrase can be *om*, the universal sound, or something that is specifically important to you, such as *peace* or *love*. With your focus on this repetitive sound, you are able to "transcend" your consciousness and become one with the universe.

Like yoga, meditation is a practice, which means it takes time to learn and it takes time to get used to. Also like yoga, if you don't like one style, you can try another. You can meditate on your own or practice with a teacher. Meditation's many benefits are worth the time investment of ten minutes a day to take yourself out of your own mind and ground yourself in the world around you.

HEALTH ISSUES
THAT RESPOND
TO GROUNDING

—

"The greatest wealth is health."

VIRGIL

The history of illness is the story of a long, slow journey with many wrong turns. One of those wrong turns was the belief that each system of the body—circulation, for example—is separate from the others. Over the last few decades, a more holistic way of treating patients has become the norm. The word *holistic* refers to the body as a complete system and the belief that health is affected by both the mind and the body.

Furthermore, researchers, doctors, and patients also recognize that seemingly unrelated causes might be tied to visible illnesses, and, conversely, visible illnesses can be treated with treatments that don't seem to have a direct connection to a symptom. For example, patients with cancer have reduced hospitalization for treatment-related problems when they participate in mind-body classes, such as yoga, tai chi, music therapy, dance therapy, and meditation. The lack of those classes has absolutely no relationship to the cause of any cancer, nor is the participation in these classes a cure, but it is clear that the participation in these practices can lead to more positive outcomes.

Because of this type of research, doctors now understand that practices such as grounding can provide benefits for patients even if no one yet completely understands the connection between the problem and the cure.

Following are some common illnesses and disorders that appear to respond well to grounding therapies.

INFLAMMATION

Our bodies are remarkable in the face of injury or illness. In order to keep ourselves in the best health, we have a system to heal, and one sign that our body is trying to heal from an injury or illness is inflammation. Inflammation can include an immediate and acute response to trauma or infection, such as the beginnings of a scab, as well as redness and swelling when you get a cut or have trauma from a fall.

There is also a low-level inflammation, sometimes called chronic or silent inflammation, that begins to fight ongoing illness, such as from a virus. The body can have a small pocket of chronic inflammation that it holds onto that begins to release toxins into the body.

For instance, let's say you need to have a root canal procedure because you have a damaged nerve in your mouth under a tooth. The pain you feel is the first sign that something is wrong. You go to the dentist, and she sees redness, a sign of infection and inflammation. You have the procedure and it is successful, but, for an unknown reason, your body still acts as if it is fighting the infection and produces an invisible inflammation response, which leaves you feeling tired and achy. This is chronic inflammation, and researchers suspect that many people with "invisible" symptoms suffer from this problem, including those with chronic fatigue, long COVID, and Lyme disease.

Fortunately, grounding appears to have very positive effects on chronic, low-level inflammation. According to a 2023 study published in *Biomedical Journal*, "Grounding provides a source of cellular restoration and energy by supporting the mitochondria or the microscopic power plants that literally provide energy to the cell." In other words, your body responds at a cellular level to being on the ground, and that energy transfer appears to decrease the overall level of inflammation, allowing the body to return to a healthier state. According to Harvard Medical School, some cancers, heart disease, diabetes, arthritis, depression, and Alzheimer's are some of the diseases now thought to be linked to chronic inflammation.

It's likely that you have, at some point, not only seen an inflammation response, such as when you bang your knee and it gets red, but also felt the inflammation response in a stressful or scary moment. You might feel your temperature rise slightly and your heart rate increase. This is called the "stress response," and it is directly related to inflammation, as well as some chronic illnesses. Chronic stress can contribute to the diseases mentioned above, as well as addiction and obesity, because stress can cause people to overeat, avoid exercise, and not sleep well.

Regulating the Inflammation Response

The thing to understand about chronic stress and inflammation is that sometimes the events that cause stress are real (such as a death in your family, moving, a breakup, or being mistreated at work) and sometimes they aren't (feeling anxious about imagined slights, for example). Either way, you need to take care of yourself and deal with not only the symptoms but also the underlying causes. That's because inflammation is only necessary when your body needs to fight disease or injury. If there is no disease or injury present, then the inflammation response is the disease itself.

To regulate this response, it helps to lie on the floor or a grounding mat, which reduces the inflammation, thus allowing the body to return to a non-inflamed state. However, it is not enough to lie on the ground in order to control and possibly reverse inflammation. Because it is a whole-body disease, you must also include a non-inflammatory diet, exercise, and, as stated above, some mind-body techniques to "tame the flame." Here are some suggestions:

1. Eat whole foods and avoid processed foods.

2. Take time away from your phone and social media.

3. Spend time in nature, including on the ground.

4. Practice savasana, or Corpse pose, i.e., lying on the ground on your back with your hands at your sides, palms facing up.

5. Move your body, including taking walks outside.

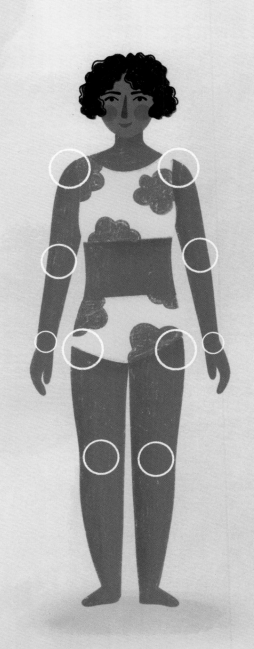

ANXIETY

According to the World Health Organization, anxiety disorders affect more than 300 million people worldwide, and it's important to know that there are highly effective treatments for them.

Although everyone's experience of anxiety is personal, the symptoms can include poor concentration, restlessness, abdominal upset, heart palpitations, trembling, a sense of impending danger or panic, and trouble sleeping. Sometimes anxiety presents with an acute attack, but other times it is more generalized, that is, you may walk around with a low-level sense of worry and dread.

If you suffer from anxiety, usually (but not always, unfortunately) you feel the panic and then create a worry in your mind to rationalize the physical feeling of anxiety. So, to succeed in overcoming anxiety, you need to recognize not only the physical symptoms but also the mental habits that contribute to the physical feelings.

Ground Yourself Away from Anxiety

There are many ways to help yourself when you have general anxiety or an anxiety attack. Although frequently a symptom is an inability to sit still, at the same time, many people who suffer from anxiety find that grounding themselves with their feet or entire bodies on the ground calms the panic. There are a few reasons this solution may help. First, it takes your focus away from the thoughts in your head. Second, grounding yourself to the floor or actual ground may help reduce the electromagnetic signals contributing to the feelings of stress.

Of all the different health issues that grounding can affect, anxiety may be the one with which it is most successful because feeling "grounded" is, in many ways, the opposite of feeling "anxious." So, although the following 3-3-3 practice is recommended here, many of the other practices suggested for other health issues in this book may also help with anxiety.

HERE'S HOW TO DO THE 3-3-3 PRACTICE:

1. Take a deep breath and look around. Identify three objects outside of your body. They can be anything: a table, a lamp, a painting, or anything else.

2. Next, identify three sounds, such as the hum of a refrigerator, the sound of the wind, and a dog barking.

3. Finally, move three body parts, such as your finger, your brow, and your feet on the floor.

4. Continue to do this until you feel calm.

Researchers believe 3-3-3 works because it takes your focus away from both your thoughts and the physical symptoms of your anxiety. Plus, it grounds you to what is outside your body.

DEPRESSION

Some say depression is anger turned inward, but really, depression is a mood disorder that almost everyone goes through at some point in their lives. The symptoms of depression, according to the National Institute of Mental Health, include feeling persistently sad, anxious, empty, or hopeless, among other negative emotions.

According to research, the best treatments for depression include talk therapy and medication, but various forms of exercise have also been shown to help. If you suffer from depression, consider committing to a workout that you enjoy. It is difficult, of course, to get out of bed when you are depressed, but there are a number of grounding activities that may help you feel strong enough to get out of bed and then strong enough to get outside and truly ground yourself.

Focus on the Present

People who feel depressed often ruminate on events from the past, often with good reason. That past event may have been painful or traumatic. The important thing to remember, though, is that the event is over. Of course, you might still be living with the fallout from that event. It's important to validate the reality of your experience and your feelings about that experience.

Nevertheless, it is also important to recognize that it is likely that you are, in the present moment, separate from that event. So, in order to ground yourself in the present, try the following exercise. It is designed to keep you in the present. The questions may seem silly and the answers obvious, but they are designed to help you transition from being immersed in your depression to being hopeful in the present.

1. Start by answering these questions: What is your name? Where do you live? How old are you? What day of the week is it? What month is it? If you are in bed, how does your bed feel? The idea is to get out of your brain, which is likely telling you things that make you feel sad, and then focus on facts that do not make you feel sad.

2. Next, see if you can sit up in your bed. Put your feet on the floor. What do you see? What noises do you hear?

3. Now, if possible, stand up, get dressed, and go outside. As you walk around your bedroom, focus not on your inner monologue, but on your steps on the floor. Notice your leg as your foot presses down and you reorganize your posture. This keeps your focus on your body. Focus on your breath.

Focus on Your Environment

Head outside for another grounding technique. Start to walk, and, while you do, notice everything around you. Ground yourself in the outdoors with your senses. If you live in a city or the suburbs, note the sounds of cars and people. Smell the air. Move your eyes around and each time you land on a different sight, such as a building or person, describe it to yourself: there's a limestone building; there's a tall man with a black coat. Grounding yourself in what's around and outside of you rather than what you're thinking and feeling inside is a good way to get out of your own head.

By the way, these are good habits to do not only when you feel depressed but also when you are happy, so that when you do feel sad, you can rely on them and not have to remind yourself to do them; they will part of your regular routine.

POST-TRAUMATIC STRESS DISORDER

According to the National Institute of Mental Health, post-traumatic stress disorder (PTSD) can occur when you have experienced a shocking event that was scary or dangerous. Although everyone needs time to process and cope with upsetting events, some people, especially if the events are ongoing or not dealt with properly, continue to suffer from symptoms long after the actual event has occurred and even if they are now safe.

Some of the symptoms of post-traumatic stress are flashbacks, recurring dreams or memories, racing heart, sweating, and panic attacks. Sometimes these symptoms arise unexpectedly, but often certain words, thoughts, and feelings can trigger the symptoms.

Ground Yourself with Meditation

Depending on your PTSD experience and your symptoms, you might want to talk to (or continue to talk to) a therapist before trying out grounding exercises. That's because people who suffer from PTSD can be triggered in unexpected ways and at unexpected times, so it's important that someone help you deal with this potential, as well as the experience if it happens.

It's helpful to read the following out loud, because the focus and the sound of your voice will help bring you out of the anxiety you may be feeling. But you can also have someone read this to you so you can close your eyes, or record the meditation and play it back so you can follow the directions.

1. Sit on the edge of a chair or couch with your feet on the floor. If possible, sit outside with your feet on the ground.

2. Place your hands on your knees, lower your shoulders away from your ears, and, if it is comfortable for you, close your eyes.

3. Breathe in through your nose for a count of three.

4. Breathe out for a count of six.

5. Repeat this breathing pattern five times.

6. Notice the way your feet feel on the ground.

7. Now, imagine there is a white light above your head and it is shining down into your body. It is traveling behind your face, down your neck, and into your shoulders. Continue to take long, slow deep breaths.

8. The white light is now floating down to fill your arms, chest, and back.

9. Picture the white light going down your spine and into your pelvis and hips, and then picture the white light moving into your legs.

10. The white light moves down your legs and into your feet, and then it connects you to the earth. The white light moves through your body from above and below, connecting you to the ground.

ADDICTION

Many of us rely on some type of distraction from our lives, such as alcohol, drugs, TV, food, or our phones. Like all of the health issues in this book, addiction is a multipronged issue, and for most people, recovery requires numerous interventions. Grounding does have a place in that recovery, as it seeks to replace your connection to your addiction with connection to the earth.

For our purposes, we're going to use cell phone addiction to describe ways in which grounding therapies can help you disconnect from your addiction. First, it's important to know that the creators smartphones and apps build in addictive qualities, including the ability to scroll. Like casinos, which block out all outside light and don't display any clocks, smartphones emit light that engages people, and many apps don't allow you to see the time while you play or scroll.

Moreover, scientists at Johns Hopkins University believe that some apps, because of the variable reinforcement of "likes" and rewards in games, keep you engaged because you believe that, at some point, you will get a dopamine hit. This "belief" is purely unconscious, but it's the idea that "If I play one more time, I'll feel better."

Dopamine is a neurotransmitter that helps us feel good when we experience something we like. It's a part of the brain's reward system. When someone "likes" your Instagram post or you bite into a chocolate chip cookie, you get a little hit of dopamine.

The problem is that, as anyone who continues to scroll (or eat cookies) knows, many people want more and more dopamine hits, and, unfortunately the more you get, the less those hits make you feel good. You know the experience. That first cookie tastes great, but that fourth or fifth cookie no longer provides a taste experience, but, instead, often makes you feel worse.

Just like endless scrolling.

There are two additional problems with these addictive behaviors. First, because the "hits" are unreliable, we go back for more in the hopes of getting the hit, and because we can't rely on it, it feeds into our need. Second, when we lose that dopamine hit, we miss it, and thus, we want it even more.

Of course, dopamine levels are not the only issues underlying addictions and addictive behaviors. Also, dopamine levels are also connected to other health issues, including depression and Parkinson's disease. Fortunately, there are other ways to get dopamine hits that are not addictive, including, of course, being outside and being grounded.

Healthy Dopamine Sources

Some of the best ways to increase dopamine without worrying about the "hit or miss" effect are listening to music, eating healthy fats, such as those found in nuts and avocados, and exercising in nature, such as taking walks, especially in sunlight.

Eat protein sources, especially those high in L-tyrosine, an amino acid, which increases the availability of dopamine. These foods include dairy products, eggs, beans, whole grains, beef, lamb, chicken, fish, and nuts. However, reducing your intake of saturated fat can also help with dopamine, so it's possible that beans and nuts are better alternatives than meats. We also know that inflammation is linked to a high intake of saturated fat. Recent research has also found that gut health is linked to neurotransmitters in the brain, so getting your L-tyrosine from yogurt and other fermented foods may be helpful in that way, too.

Getting natural sunlight and enough sleep have an important relationship with dopamine. The correct level of dopamine promotes wakefulness in a person's sleep-wake cycle.

JET LAG

If you fly from New York to Paris—west to east, five or six time zones depending on the time of year—it's likely that jet lag will bother you for at least two days. That's because your body is on a relatively stable circadian rhythm of twenty-four hours and if you take good care of yourself, it's likely that you go to sleep at a relatively regular hour and wake up at roughly the same time each morning.

Ever since the beginning of the air travel age, people have looked for ways to stop jet lag from ruining their vacations, including taking medications with serious side effects. Fortunately, though, grounding and sunlight seem to be both the most effective and the safest way to reduce this problem.

According to a 2023 study published in *Biomedical Journal*, the circadian rhythm is influenced by light and the earth's electromagnetic fields. Flying in a plane and disrupting your typical circadian rhythm can increase inflammation, fatigue, and flu-like symptoms.

To counteract these problems, researchers are studying grounding, and, at least preliminarily, it appears that grounding is effective in reducing the likelihood of feeling jet lag. Therefore, aside from avoiding alcohol and trying to sleep on the plane, as well as spending a few days before your trip trying to gradually adjust to the new time zone, you can combine grounding and light exposure to center yourself in your new location.

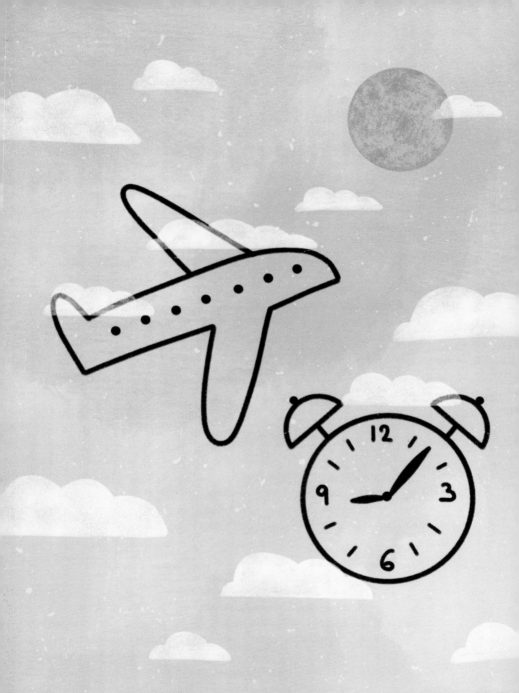

Grounding When You Arrive

First, of course, you'll get to where you're staying. Then, as early in the day as possible, walk to a park (lots of them in Paris) or the beach (if you're not in a city, but somewhere more peaceful), and take off your shoes. With the sun on your face (we hope!), stand on the earth or in the water. Just relax there for twenty minutes, making sure you let your toes wiggle in the grass or the sand.

Grounding increases the alpha waves (which have a frequency of 7.5Hz) in the brain. Alpha waves are present during deep relaxation and meditation, and they give us access to our imagination, memory, learning, and concentration. These waves help improve sleep and normalize the secretion of cortisol and melatonin.

Later, after a fun day of, we hope, either walking or swimming (so you stay in touch with earth or water), consider sleeping on a grounding mat placed on the floor. Doing this balances levels of cortisol, which helps synchronize your circadian rhythm.

If you're in a hotel room and can't wait to get into that nice comfy bed, spending twenty minutes on the grounding mat will be enough to reconnect you to the earth.

GROUNDING
LOCATIONS

—

"Travel makes one modest.
You see what a tiny place you occupy
in the world."

GUSTAVE FLAUBERT

If you've traveled, whether to a park on the opposite side of the world or a beach in a nearby state, you've probably had the experience of finding yourself somewhere and realizing that it just "felt good." There are some places on earth that have anecdotally brought peace to people for hundreds of years. It turns out that there may be some science to back up why certain places have become so meaningful to millions of travelers, and that science points to grounding.

THE SEVEN EARTH CHAKRAS

Before we explain the locations of the earth chakras, let's first understand the body chakras. In Hindu and Buddhist yoga traditions, the word *chakra*, which means "circle" or "wheel," refers to energy centers in the body. These centers aren't literal within the body. Instead, they correspond to a location in which nerve bundles and organs play a role in your physical health. (*Chakra*, by the way, is pronounced "chuhk-ra" with a soft "sh" and a soft "uh" sound in the first syllable.)

Within this tradition of thinking, your health is somewhat dependent on keeping your chakras open and balanced. When you are in poor health, the reason might be because your chakras are blocked. There are seven main chakras, and each one is related to an invisible line of energy that runs from the base of your spine to above your head. Each chakra is associated with a yoga pose, a color (in the order of the rainbow), and an emotion.

Muladhara
base of the spine/sphincter
red

This is called the root chakra, and it is your foundation for life. When it is stable, you feel grounded and secure. When it is out of balance, you feel unmoored and frightened. Practice Tree pose to feel stable.

TREE

1. Start in Mountain pose: Feet hip width apart, core engaged, and feet pressed firmly into the ground. Find a spot on the ground to look at; this will help with your balance.

2. On an inhale, raise your arms without bringing your shoulders to your ears. You can bring your hands together. While doing this, bend your left leg and bring your left foot to rest on your right leg. You can instead rest the toes on the ground and put your left heel on your right foot if balance is a problem for you.

3. Exhale but keep the balance in your legs. If you feel unsteady, engage your core. Don't worry about swaying. Trees sway.

4. Hold this posture for about 30 seconds.

5. Switch to the other side.

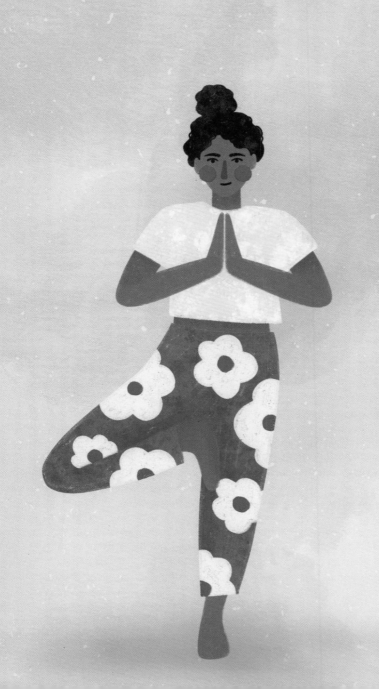

Svadhisthana
sacral spine
orange

The sacral chakra is the life force, related to sexual and creative energy. When stable, you feel in touch with your emotions and with others. When blocked, you feel disconnected from others. When you practice Garland pose, you open this chakra and energize your sexuality and relationships.

GARLAND

1. Stand with feet far apart, toes pointed out, heels toward each other, as if you're in second position in ballet. Bring your knees over your feet; you should be able to see your big toes.

2. Keep your core engaged and shoulders down.

3. Begin to squat, keeping thighs apart, and bring hands together. If you can, you can rest your upper arms against your thighs.

4. Hold this posture for 30 seconds.

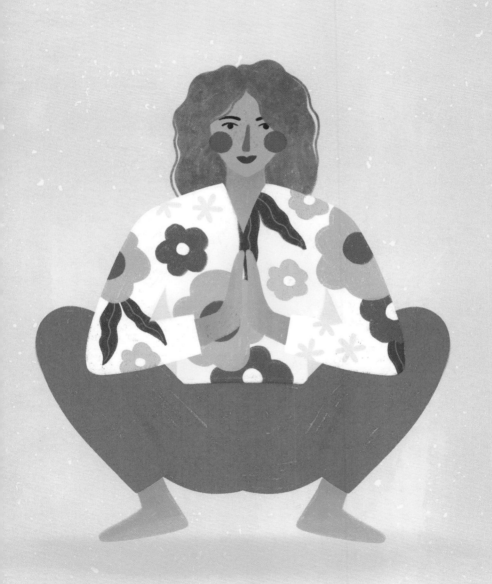

Manipura
navel
yellow

This is known as the solar plexus chakra, and it governs your stomach area. When it's in balance, you feel confident. When it's out of balance, you may have digestive issues related to your emotions. To help energize this chakra, practice Boat pose.

BOAT

1. Sit on floor with knees bent, feet on floor. Be sure your back is straight, shoulders away from ears, lengthen the chest.

2. Begin to lean back while raising your knees, to balance on your sit bones.

3. If you can, begin to straighten your legs. You may need to put your hands under your thighs.

4. If possible, lean back with legs straight, so you are making a "V" shape.

5. Inhale and exhale for a few breaths.

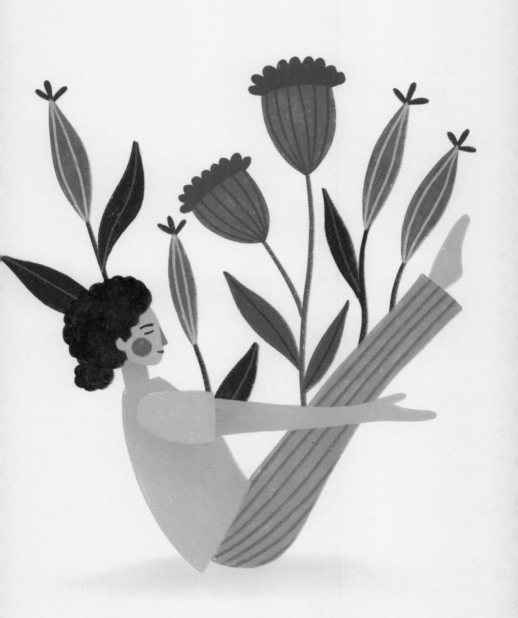

Anahata
heart
green

Located in your chest, around your heart, this chakra relates to your ability to love in all its manifestations. When it is blocked, you may feel lonely or insecure. Practicing Camel pose will open your chest and give you a chance to practice bringing your breath and energy to this part of your body.

CAMEL

1. Kneel on floor with knees together and ankles together, hips lifted off legs, and toes tucked under feet.

2. Keeping your core engaged, inhale and left up, bringing your arms over your head.

3. Start to reach back, trying to bring your hands to your heels into a backbend. Keep lifting your chest and lengthening your neck.

4. This is a tough pose. If it's too hard, stand and lean into a backbend, with hands on your lower back. Imagine that you want to be longer, not crunched.

5. Hold the backbend for 30 seconds. Come up slowly.

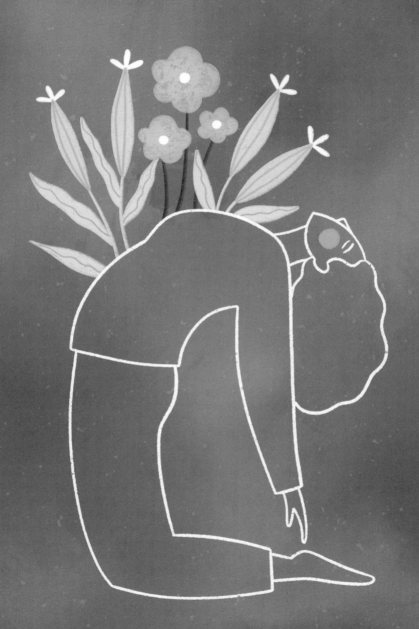

Vishuddha
throat
blue

This is known as the throat chakra because it is located in your throat. This chakra has to do with your ability to communicate verbally, and when it is blocked you may have trouble expressing your truth. To help support this chakra, you can do Nine-Count Pranayama Breathing pose.

NINE-COUNT PRANAYAMA BREATHING

Many "hot" yoga classes begin with this sequence. It's a great way to center yourself to start class. Also, it relaxes the entire upper body so that you can breathe deeply through class. Focus on counting slowly while you do this.

1. Stand with your feet parallel, toes and heels touching, core engaged, and shoulders away from ears.

2. Interlace your fingers under your chin and bring your forearms and elbows together in front of your upper body. Stay relaxed. Look forward.

3. Take three counts to inhale while keeping your hands together and raising your elbows while bending your head back, gently. Your knuckles stay under your chin. Bring your breath to the back of the throat.

4. While your head is gently bent back, begin to exhale slowly on a count of three, while bringing your elbows together.

5. On the final count of three, come back to the start position. Do this nine more times. If you want to be traditional, do another set of ten.

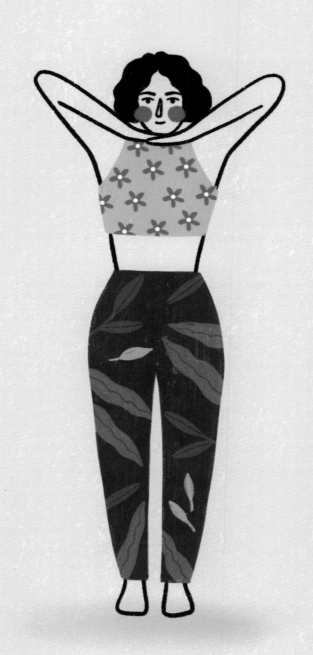

Ajna
between the eyes
purple

This is known as the third eye chakra because it is located between your eyes. You can thank this chakra for a strong gut instinct. That's because the third eye is responsible for intuition. It's also linked to imagination. When this chakra is blocked, you may feel foggy or indecisive. Viparita Karani or Legs Up the Wall Pose connects your energy to the earth's energy.

VIPARITA KARANI OR LEGS UP THE WALL POSE

Many yogis consider this the most relaxing yoga pose. It activates the relaxation response, which is a state of deep rest that changes your physical and emotional response to stress. When you can access the relaxation response, your heart rate and blood pressure remain low, and you can breathe deeply.

When doing this pose, you can raise your legs onto a couch, bed, or chair instead of a wall.

1. Lie with your rear end close to a wall as possible..

2. Roll onto your back and, as you do this, bring your legs against the wall, scrunching your rear end to the wall.

3. Your upper body should remain on the floor, arms by your sides.

4. Let yourself relax into the floor and let the floor support you.

5. Lie this way for 10 minutes, breathing deeply, eyes closed. If you want, put a weighted eye pillow on your eyes.

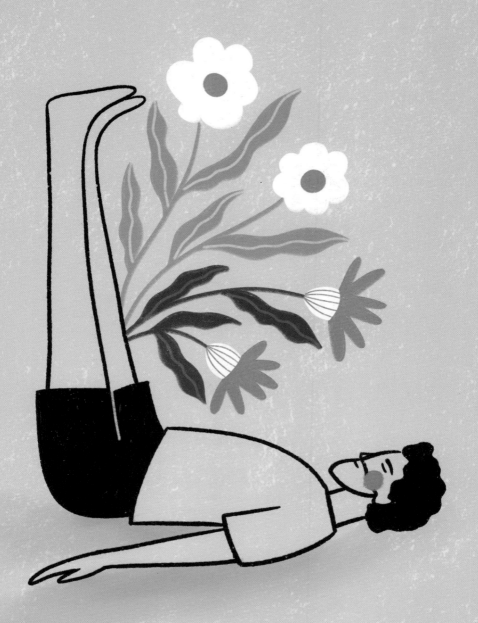

Sahasrara
crown of the head
white

The crown chakra is located at the top of your head. It represents your spiritual connection to yourself, others, and the universe. It also plays a role in your life's purpose. When this chakra is blocked, you may feel detached from yourself, others, or your higher purpose. Easy pose is designed to bring all your energy to your highest self.

EASY POSE

1. This is a common sitting position, and has a lot of names outside of yoga, such as Criss Cross Apple-sauce. In yoga, though, you want to make sure you aren't slouched and really feel the ground beneath you.

2. Be sure to cross your legs at your shins, and, if possible, put each foot under the opposite knee with the toes pointing forward. The outer edges of your feet should rest on the floor.

3. Sit in this posture for 30 seconds to two minutes, being sure to keep your shoulders away from your ears and your abs engaged. It's "easy" because you are letting the ground hold you, but it's still a posture you need to "hold."

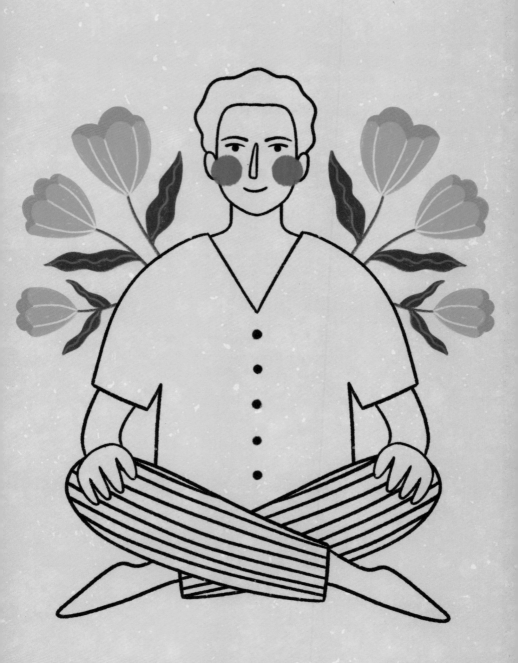

Meanwhile, the earth also has chakra points, and they relate to emotions, health, and spirituality, just like the body chakras. Earth's chakras are found along the ley lines of the planet. Sites along these lines support the idea of special magnetic energy in some locations. This thinking is in line with the discovery of the Schumann resonances. According to NASA, there are electromagnetic waves between the earth's surface and a boundary about 60 miles (97 km) above earth. Of course, there are always lightning and thunderstorms somewhere on the planet, as well as other charged particles in the atmosphere. These waves are at an extremely low frequency, yet are measurable. They correspond to the seasons, solar activity, and other weather-related phenomena.

This magnetic energy is most noticeable at certain locations on earth. Not surprisingly, many of them have become sacred locations for various populations, and, ultimately, significant travel destinations. It's important to travel to these destinations with a sense of reverence, being sure to treat the earth respectfully. Going to these places isn't like traveling to man-made spectacles such as the Eiffel Tower. These are natural locations that are believed to hold healing energy, and a few of them, such as Mount Shasta, Lake Titicaca, Uluru, Stonehenge, and the Great Pyramid of Giza, are UNESCO World Heritage sites. When you visit, you'll want to take off your shoes!

Mount Shasta, California — Muladhara

Indigenous peoples, including the Shasta, Klamath, Pit, Modoc, and Wintu tribes, lived for many years around this 14,162-foot dormant volcano in the Cascade range of California. Mount Shasta has a double peak. It last erupted in 1786, but the area is geographically active, as its tectonic plates shift and there are recorded earthquakes. Mount Shasta's glaciers feed the McCloud, Sacramento, and Shasta rivers. John Muir wrote, "When I first caught sight of Mount Shasta over the braided folds of the Sacramento Valley, my blood turned to wine, and I have not been weary since."

For many people, mountains are a reassuring vista, as you can see them from far away. You can also hike up mountains and although you shouldn't do this barefoot, of course, being on a path up a mountain engages you with the earth. In addition, you see the world differently from a mountain. Often, when people feel disconnected from themselves, they head to the mountains in order to get a literally different point of view. You might feel "on top of the world" when you're on a mountain because that shift from seeing the world at its base versus seeing the landscape from above encourages you to look at your life with a wider and more generous perspective.

Mountains illustrate the ageless wisdom of the earth. The fact that they are wide at the bottom and reach high into the sky serve as a metaphor for people. They remind us of the old saying that "children need roots and wings." Mountains are connected to the root chakra, as their wide base is rooted to the earth and provides a sense of stability from which to grow.

Mountain Meditation

If you feel stuck and want to make changes in your life, but are having a hard time taking those first steps, consider visiting Mount Shasta or a mountain near you. It likely won't be as tall as Mount Shasta, but you can still take advantage of the energy of a new perspective.

This meditation is designed to help you feel grounded while inviting change and progress into your life.

1. When you are in a safe location, i.e., not climbing on a rocky footpath, but instead somewhere steady with a view, consider taking off your shoes.

2. Stand in Mountain pose, feel parallel, with the bases of your big toes touching and your heels slightly apart. Engage your abdominals and gently tuck your pelvis so it is balanced between your hips. Breathe deeply without raising your shoulders toward your ears. Relax your arms, letting them drift away from your torso, and let your palms face forward.

3. Take long, slow, deep breaths. On an inhale, imagine your breath going toward your feet, grounding yourself to the earth beneath you. On an exhale, begin to image your future. What is it you want? When you inhale again, bring your breath back to your feet and where you are right now. On the exhale, again, imagine your future. Do this for as long as you need to. Remember, it's a tool to help you descend the mountain as a slightly different person.

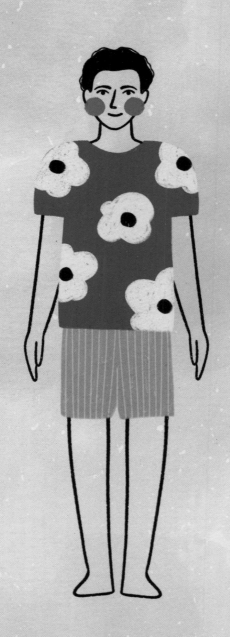

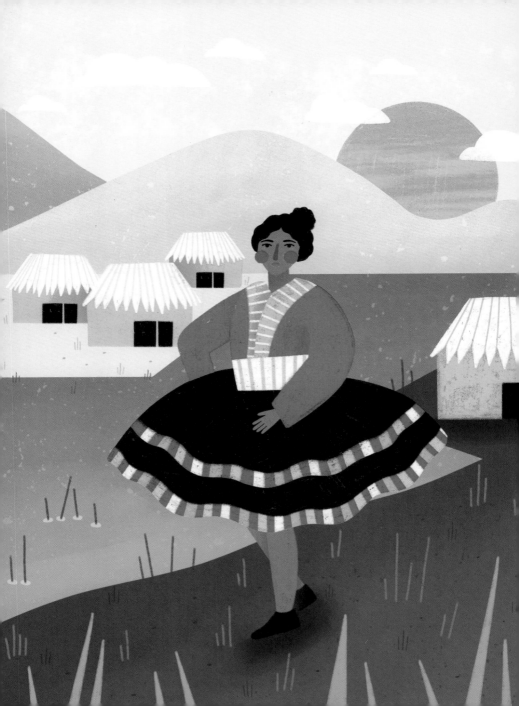

Lake Titicaca, South America — Svadhisthana

A freshwater lake in the Andes Mountains, Lake Titicaca sits on the border between Bolivia and Peru. It is the world's largest navigable body of water. Although no one is sure, many historians think it is the birthplace of the Incas, because there are ruins around the lake. This ancient lake is thought to be three million years old. It is famously still and calm, reflective of the skies. The wetlands and animals around the lake are as significant as the lake itself. While its original meaning is unknown, today the word *titicaca* translates to "mountain of the puma" or "stone puma." The Incas believed it was the birthplace of the sun.

The gift of Lake Titicaca and the second chakra is to feel your sexuality and creativity in balance. That is to say, this isn't a chakra of promiscuity or uncontrolled expression. When your second chakra is in balance, you trust your intuition and feel open to opportunities, but you are not wild or uninhibited.

Dance!

One of the best ways to unblock your second chakra is to dance. Put on some music and let your body respond without judgment. Some dance moves that are especially connected to the sacral chakra are the twist and the hula, which rotate your hips. If you aren't comfortable dancing, consider playing with a hula hoop or even just circling your hips in both directions with your feet apart. Other options are squats and pliés, but try to keep music on while you do them so you can respond to the rhythm.

Uluru, Australia — Manipura

The world's largest monolith, Uluru is in central Australia and reaches a height 2,831 feet (863 m). It is 2.2 miles (3.5 km) long by 1.5 miles (2.4 km) wide, with a circumference of 5.8 miles (9.3 km). The rock is sandstone and feldspar. At sunset, the rock looks like it's on fire and appears orange-red. The top and bottom look different from each other. The lower slopes are fluted due to erosion, while the top has basins. There are caves at its base that contain carvings and paintings made by Australia's indigenous peoples.

The solar plexus chakra is your physical energy center. All chakras have specific energy, but the solar plexus is your core. When your third chakra is in balance, you have the energy and focus to work toward your goals without trying to hurt anyone or gain power over others. Your power is for yourself, and so you will feel free and strong, just like this enormous monolith.

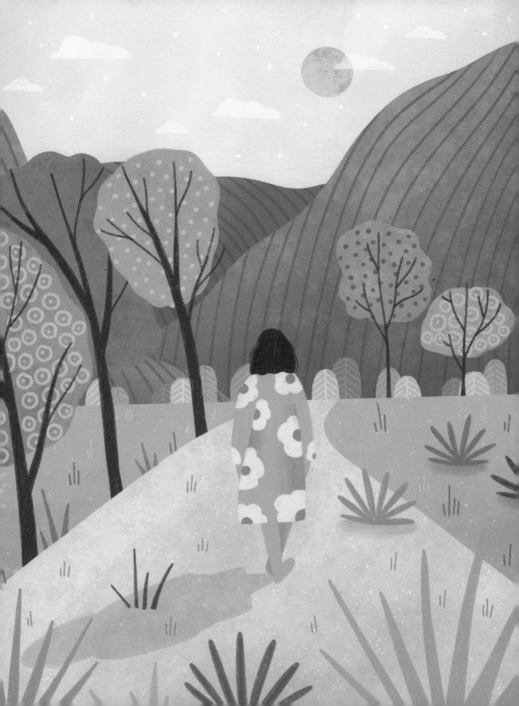

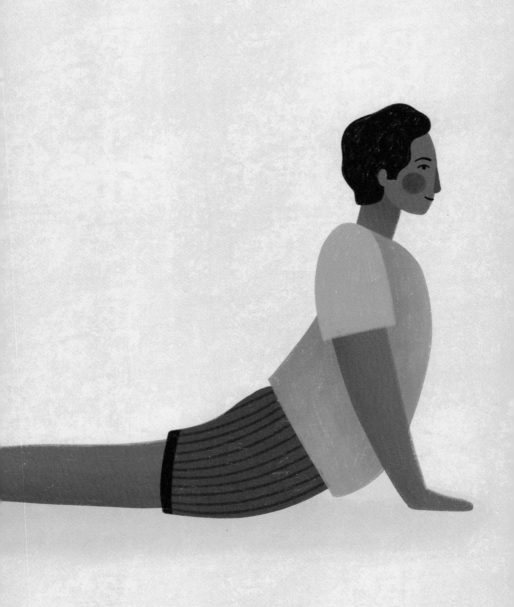

Cobra Pose

Cobra pose lifts and strengthens the solar plexus.

1. Lie with your belly on the floor, palms on the floor directly under your shoulders. Place your elbows alongside your body and make sure your shoulders are pulled away from your ears and your torso is elongated against the floor.

2. On an inhale, slowly straighten your elbows to 45 degrees while you lift your head, neck, and shoulders. Keep your lower torso against the floor and your legs straight. Your neck should be neutral.

3. On an exhale, lower your upper body and turn your head to one side against the floor.

4. Do this five more times, turning your head to the opposite side each time.

Glastonbury Tor, England — Anahata

A tor is a freestanding rock outcrop that seems to appear by itself without other rocks nearby. The word *tor* was first used by the Welsh and often refers to a rock on the top of a hill in the English countryside, but there are tors all over the world. Originally the word meant "castle," but not in terms of a building. Nevertheless, the Glastonbury Tor is a tower that sits on a hill, and it is prominent in Celtic mythology and the stories of King Arthur. There are also abbey ruins at the site.

Glastonbury Tor is said to be the heart chakra of the earth. One reason is that for many years the tor was the center of many Druid priestess rituals. Those who believe in ley lines think two converge at Glastonbury, very close to the supposed gravesite of King Arthur and Guinevere. Standing at this site is said to bring on deep feelings of love. Some people believe that Joseph of Arimathea is also buried here, as he brought the Holy Grail to this site. This is, of course, part of the Arthurian legends.

To start every day with an open heart, try doing the Sun Salutation every morning.

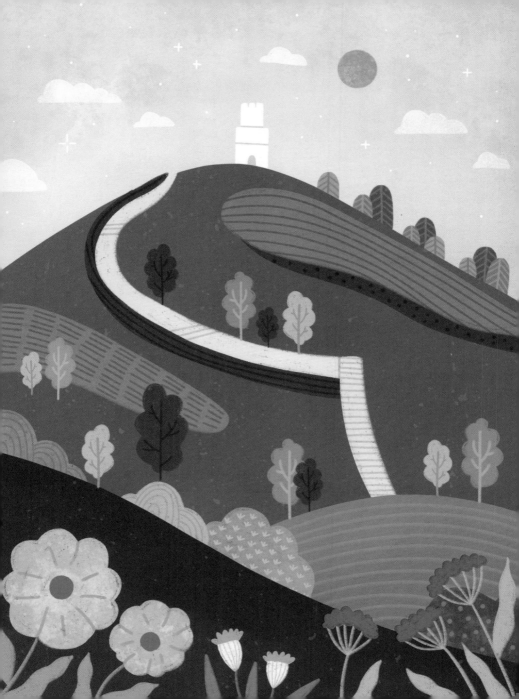

Sun Salutation

There are three Sun Salutation variations in Ashtanga yoga, and, ideally, you will do each three times (A, A, A, B, B, B, C, C, C). Doing these sequences is a wonderful way to move from sleep to wakefulness. Keep your yoga mat by your bed so you can start your practice easily. It will take about fifteen minutes. Don't rush the first sequences or push through the poses, because your body needs time to stretch.

Sun Salutation is done as a flowing sequence (vinyasa), so you'll move from one pose to the next. If you have a yoga mat, begin at the top because you will move down the length of the mat with the flow. The flow of postures matches the breath to the movement. Don't rush. The goal isn't to finish quickly, but to take deep breaths and relax into the postures. You'll see "inhale" and "exhale" at the beginning of each pose. This doesn't mean you should hold your breath at any time. You will also breathe while you're in the postures.

Sun Salutation A

1.   Begin in Mountain pose (Tadasana), arms by your sides, feet hip-width apart, and chin parallel to the floor.

2.   On an inhale, begin to flow into Exalted Mountain, bringing your arms out and above your head. Touch your fingers.

3.   On an exhale, come down into Standing Forward Fold (Uttanasana), hands to floor. If you can't touch the floor, you can use blocks.

4.   Inhale and come into Half-Forward Fold (Ardha Uttanasana) with a flat back, feet parallel to the floor, fingers on your shins or blocks.

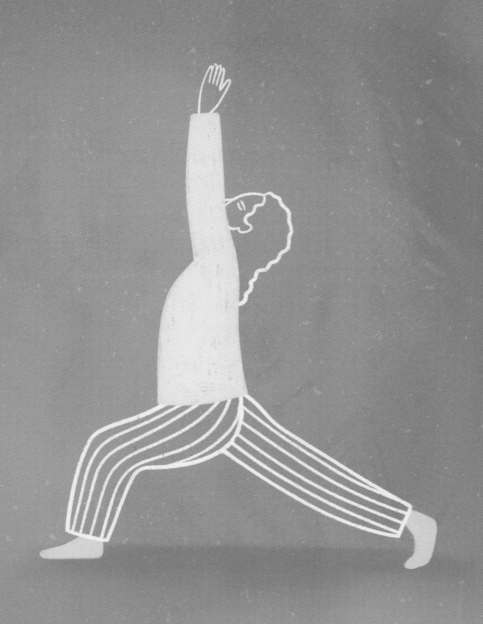

5. Exhale and step back into Plank, then lower to the floor in Four-Limbed Staff pose (Chaturanga). Make sure your wrists are under your elbows and shoulders and that you are maintaining a neutral spine. The goal is to hover on your fingers and toes just slightly above the floor, but that may be difficult. Consider coming down to the floor very slowly, as if you were doing a reverse push-up. Be sure to engage your abdominals and keep your neck and back straight.

6. On an inhale, come into Upward-Facing Dog (Urdhva Mukha Svanasana). Roll onto the tops of your feet and straighten your arms. Try to lift your thighs away from the floor as you lift your chest. This is a bigger backbend than Cobra, but they are similar.

7. Exhale and come into Downward-Facing Dog (Adho Mukha Svanasana). Uncurl your toes and extend through your feet, bringing your hips up and flattening your back as if to make the shape of an inverted V. Your arms are straight. Look between your feet and hold for five breaths.

8. Now, you're going to return to the starting pose. On an inhale, step into Half-Forward Fold (Ardha Utta-nasana). On an exhale, drop back down into Standing Forward Fold (Uttanasana). Inhale and rise back up to Mountain pose (Tadasana).

9. Repeat the sequence twice for a total of three times.

Sun Salutation B

1. Stand at the top of your mat in Mountain pose (Tadasana), arms by your sides, feet hip-width apart, and chin parallel to the floor.

2. On an inhale, bend your knees and come into Chair pose (Utkatasana); this looks like a squat, as if you are sitting in a chair. Bring your arms up, keeping your abdominals engaged and your spine long.

3. On an exhale, and in one slow movement, straighten your legs and bend forward to come into Standing Forward Fold (Uttanasana). Bring your hands to the floor or blocks.

4. On an inhale, come into Half-Forward Fold (Ardha Uttanasana) with a flat back, feet parallel to the floor, fingers on your shins or blocks.

5. Exhale and come into Plank, then lower into Four-Limbed Staff pose (Chaturanga Dandasana). Make sure your wrists are under your elbows and shoulders and that you are maintaining a neutral spine. The goal is to hover on your fingers and toes just slightly above the floor, but that may be difficult. Consider coming down to the floor very slowly, as if you were doing a reverse push-up. Be sure to engage your abdominals and keep your neck and back straight.

6. Inhale and roll your feet so the tops are against the floor to come into Upward-Facing Dog (Urdhva Mukha Svanasana). Straighten your arms and try to lift your thighs away from the floor, abdominals engaged, shoulders away from ears. You are stretching your chest and letting your back gently curve.

7. Exhale into Downward-Facing Dog (Adho Mukha Svanasana). Put your feet flat against the floor if you can (heels may be a little raised) and come into an inverted V position. Hold for five breaths, using the breath energy to deepen the pose.

8. Now, inhale to come into Warrior 1 (Virabhadrasana) on the right side. To do this, step your right foot between your hands and turn your left foot out slightly. Your right heel should be aligned with the arch of your left foot. Bend your right knee and lift your torso upright, opening your chest to the side, as you straighten your arms out from your shoulders.

9. To move to the other side, go through a vinyasa of Four-Legged Staff pose (Chaturanga Dandasana) on an exhale, Upward-Facing Dog (Urdhva Mukha Svanasana) on an inhale, and Downward-Facing Dog (Adho Mukha Svanasana) on an exhale.

10. Now, on an inhale, come into Warrior 1 (Virabhadrasana 1) on the left side. Your left foot is forward, right foot angled behind you. The left heel is aligned with the right arch. Bend your left knee and lift your torso upright, opening your chest to the side, as you straighten your arms out from your shoulders.

11. Exhale and come through your vinyasa again: Four-Legged Staff (Chaturanga Dandasana) on an exhale, Upward-Facing Dog (Urdhva Mukha Svanasana) on an inhale, and Downward-Facing Dog (Adho Mukha Svanasana) on an exhale.

12. To end the sequence, inhale to move forward on your mat, then exhale and come into Standing Forward Fold (Uttanasana).

13. Inhale and come into Half-Forward Fold (Ardha Uttanasana). Exhale as you move into an inhale and return to Chair pose (Utkatasana).

14. Finally, inhale and rise to Mountain pose (Tadasana).

15. Repeat the sequence twice for a total of three times.

Sun Salutation C

1. Stand at the top of your mat in Mountain pose (Tadasana), arms by your sides, feet hip-width apart, and chin parallel to the floor.

2. On an inhale, bend your knees and come into Chair pose (Utkatasana); this looks like a squat, as if you are sitting in a chair. Bring your arms up, keeping your abdominals engaged and your spine long.

3. On an exhale, and in one slow movement, straighten your legs and bend forward to come into Standing Forward Fold (Uttanasana). Bring your hands to the floor or blocks.

4. On an inhale, come into Half-Forward Fold (Ardha Uttanasana), with your back flat and parallel to the floor, fingers on your shins or on blocks. Return to Standing Forward Fold (Uttanasana).

5. Exhale and come into Low Lunge pose (Anjanayasana) on the right side. Step your left foot back and lower your left knee to the floor. The right knee is bent. Now inhale and raise your torso, reaching your arms up, shoulders away from your ears. You should feel a slight backbend.

6. Transition to the floor with the Knees/Chest/Chin variation: Come into Plank pose and as you exhale and lower your knees, chest, and chin to the floor. Then come fully down, hands under your shoulders.

7. On an inhale, come into Cobra pose (Bhujangasana). Gently straighten your arms a little (but not all the way) while your hips and thighs press gently into the floor. Lengthen your torso from head to feet, shoulders away from your ears.

8. Exhale and come into Downward-Facing Dog (Adho Mukha Svanasana), the inverted V.

9. Now move into Low Lunge (Anjanayasana) on the left side. Step your right foot back and lower your right knee to the floor. The left knee is bent. Now inhale and raise your torso, reaching your arms up, shoulders away from your ears. You should feel a slight backbend.

10. Transition to the floor with the Knees/Chest/Chin variation: Come into Plank pose and as you exhale, lower your knees, chest, and chin to the floor. Then come fully down, hands under your shoulders.

11. On an inhale, come into Cobra pose (Bhujangasana). Gently straighten your arms a little (but not all the way) while your hips and thighs press gently into the floor. Lengthen your torso from head to feet, shoulders away from your ears.

12. Exhale and come into Downward-Facing Dog (Adho Mukha Svanasana), the inverted V.

13. Now, you're going to return to the starting pose. Inhale to move forward on your mat, and then exhale and come into Standing Forward Fold (Uttanasana).

14. Inhale and come into Half-Forward Fold (Ardha Uttanasana). On an exhale, drop back down into Standing Forward Fold (Uttanasana).

15. Inhale and rise back up to Mountain pose (Tadasana).

16. Repeat the sequence twice for a total of three times.

Mount of Olives, Mount Sinai, and the Great Pyramid of Giza, the Middle East — Vishuddha

The area that includes the Mount of Olives, Mount Sinai, and the Great Pyramid of Giza is associated with the throat chakra, which, when open, is expressive and communicates your truth. The Mount of Olives is near Jerusalem while Mount Sinai and the Great Pyramid are in Egypt. These three locations are connected by straight lines that form a triangle.

Important to both Jews and Christians, the Mount of Olives is a ridge just outside Old Jerusalem. It no longer has olive trees, and its ownership has been in dispute for generations between Jordan and Israel. People of all religions come to see this beautiful spot with an amazing view of the Temple Mount, the valley of Hinnom, and the desert. There is a Russian Orthodox church, a Lutheran church, and other religious landmarks, as well as a Jewish cemetery, which has been used since the beginning of Jewish history, although much of it has been destroyed in various wars.

Mount Sinai, which is on the Sinai Peninsula in Egypt, is just one of the locations that scholars believe may have been where Moses received the Ten Commandments. Like the other chakra sites, its rocks are made of granite and feldspar, likely due to volcanoes in the very long ago past. It is almost 8,000 feet (2.4 km) tall. Mount Sinai is meaningful to Jews, Christians, and Muslims, as all three recognize Moses as a prophet. Significant historical events in all three religions—not just related to Moses—occurred on or around Mount Sinai, including that it is the site of Saint Catherine's Monastery, the longest inhabited Christian monastery. Archeologists have found ancient biblical manuscripts in its libraries.

Finally, this chakra encompasses Giza, the third largest city in Egypt and the site of the Great Pyramids, smaller pyramids, and the Great Sphinx. Located on the west bank of the Nile, it is a suburb of Cairo. The sphinx is considered a guardian of temples and tombs and is associated with riddles in ancient mythology.

Fish Pose

To unblock the throat chakra, yogis practice Fish pose (Matsayasana), which opens the front of the neck. This pose can be a strain for some people, so you can do it with a blanket under your neck and head or you can do it sitting without leaning on your head. The goal is to lift your head up so your neck and throat are open.

1. Lie on your back, soles of the feet on the floor, arms by your sides, palms facing down.

2. Lift your hips and slide your hands under your lower back, with your palms supporting your lower back.

3. Inhale and bend your elbows while you bring your head up to rest the crown of your head against the floor; lift your chest. You should feel the front of your neck open as your upper body rests on your arms and shoulders.

4. Hold this pose for five breaths.

5. To come out of the pose, uncurl gently and return to lying flat on the floor.

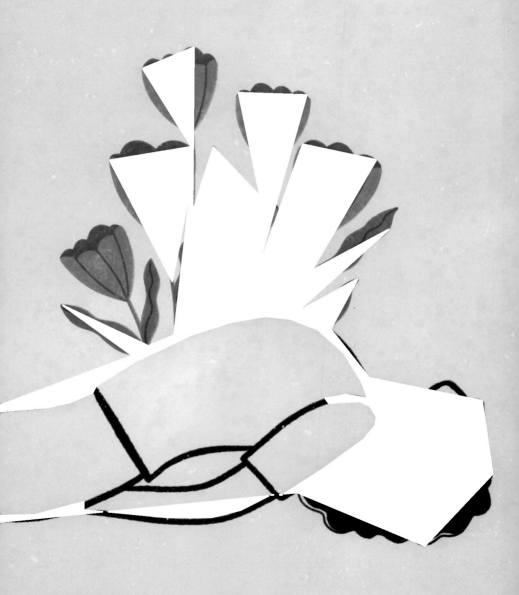

The Third Eye, No Fixed Location — Ajna

Intuition, sixth sense . . . whatever you want to call it, your third eye both has a physical location and doesn't. Physically, the third eye is located between your two eyes and slightly higher. This third eye can't "see" visually, but it senses or understands the world in a deeper, more meaningful way.

The third eye is truly electromagnetic. In fact, researchers have theorized that one reason animals respond early to earthquakes and other natural phenomena is that they sense a disturbance in the electromagnetic field. Their "magnet" is at the third eye location.

Meanwhile, on earth, the third eye chakra moves its location depending on geographical age. The third eye chakra is associated with being in tune with yourself, others, and nature.

Child's Pose

Child's pose (Balasana) supports the third eye chakra because it is a calming posture with your third eye on the floor. This spot stimulates the vagus nerve, which encourages a relaxation response.

1. Start on your hands and knees in Tabletop position, with your weight balanced between your arms and lower legs, abdominals engaged.

2. On an exhale, open your knees and sit back, bringing your torso down to the floor, elongating your arms and letting your toes touch.

3. Rest your torso on the floor, relax your shoulders, jaw, and eyes, and let your forehead rest on the floor. If this is too strenuous, you can rest your forehead on a towel or block.

4. Continue to inhale and exhale slowly.

5. Come out of the post gently.

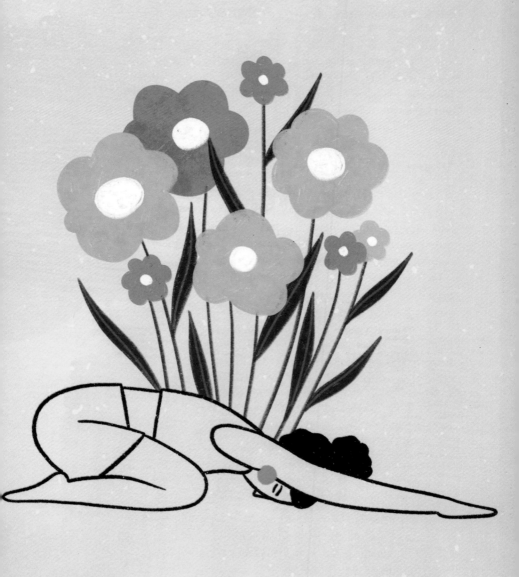

Mount Kailash, Tibet — Sahasrara

Called the "roof" of the world, Mount Kailash is located in Tibet and is one of the highest Himalayan mountains at close to 22,000 feet (6.7 km). It represents the crown chakra, which is located at the top of and above your head, connecting your body to the divine and the universe. It is the final chakra, and when it's in balance, you let go of your ego.

Savasana

To stimulate the final chakra, you will practice Corpse pose (Savasana). Remember that yoga was originally developed as a way to prepare for meditation, to help practitioners get out their excess energy in order to then sit still. It is in stillness that we fully connect with the world outside of ourselves. Not surprisingly, it is sometimes difficult for people to quiet their body and mind. Often people say that Savasana is the most challenge posture. Because you aren't moving, you might feel colder than you do during the rest of your yoga practice, so consider wearing socks and putting a blanket over you. You will breathe gently throughout this posture, but you don't link your breath with any movement.

1. Lie on your back. Let your legs gently fall open. Let your arms rest at your sides, slightly away from your body.

2. Allow your body to relax into the floor and close your eyes. Breathe slowly and gently. Consider staying like this for five to ten minutes (you may want to set a timer). You may fall asleep. That is fine.

3. To come out of the pose, open your eyes, wiggle your toes and fingers, and then stretch your arms. Roll onto your right side and push yourself up to come into a seated posture.

4. Roll your head, circle your shoulders, and stretch your body gently.

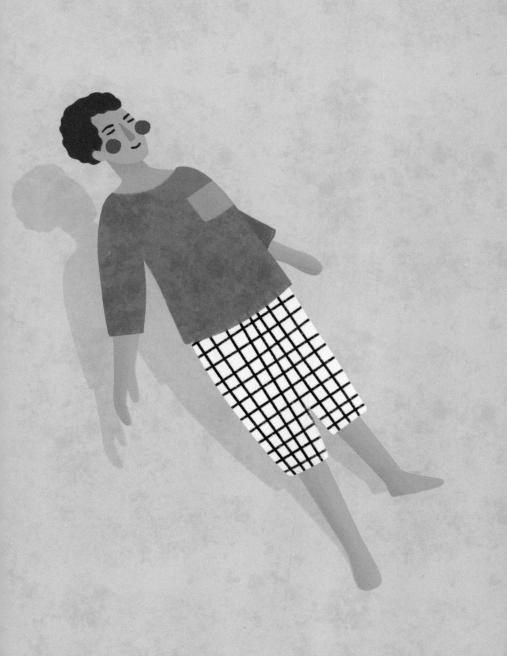

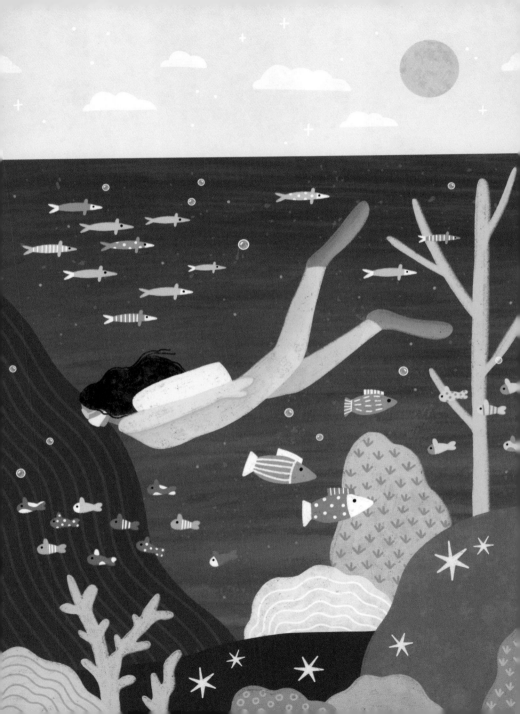

GROUNDING LOCATIONS THROUGHOUT THE WORLD

You don't have to travel to the seven earth chakras in order to reap the benefits of grounding and aligning your chakras. There are many places around the world that have drawn people for centuries because of their healing and grounding properties.

Sedona, Arizona

Let's just start with a list of the natural elements that make Sedona a truly one-of-a-kind place on Earth: First, the skies overhead are a Dark Sky Park, so you can see an abundance of stars due to a lack of artificial light interrupting this stunning experience. Second, the town has energy vortices, which are swirling centers of electromagnetic energy that humans can feel, but not see. Third, the landscape of red rocks and evergreens looks and feels magical, often immediately bringing a sense of calm to visitors. It is both a desert and a forest.

Geologists know that over millennia, rivers carve into the rocks and land, creating canyons. This takes millions of years, of course. Sedona is the southern end of a canyon, and the town was settled at the bottom with the high rocks surrounding the buildings. It's two hours away from the Grand Canyon, but has beautiful canyons all its own. Yes, it is still crowded and some locations require passes and don't allow individual cars to park at trailheads in order to reduce traffic, but these rules protect nature from people.

One of the reasons Sedona is so shockingly beautiful is that although much of it looks like a desert, the landscape includes features such as Oak Creek Canyon, which has many trees and much water. There is a true juxtaposition of landscapes in one location. The orange and red colors of the canyon formations are considered by many to stimulate creativity and a sense of peacefulness to those who unplug and take in the beauty. The red sandstone often appears to glow orange when the sun rises and sets. The Sedona landscape is a chaparral, a biome with evergreen shrubs and small trees and a mild, Mediterranean climate.

There are many famous sandstone formations in and around Sedona, including Wilson Mountain, Bell Rock, and Capitol Butte. Around Sedona are equally magical water sites, such as Seven Sacred Pools. Although no one can scientifically quantify religious experiences, because of its beauty and energy vortices, which are only beginning to be measured, inhabitants of Sedona and its many visitors believe it is a place where people experience grounding, or transformational moments that connect them to their place on earth.

Although all of Sedona is considered to be an energy vortex, it has specific places where the energy seems most vibrational. Of course, these metaphysical feelings correspond to the beautiful locations. Airport Mesa and Cathedral Canyon seem to radiate with their own energy, as do some of the other famous buttes, rocks, and canyons.

In no particular order of importance, the first specific energy vortex site is Bell Rock. You can actually hike up Bell Rock, although it is more of a scramble than a walk. Mountain bikers love it, too. It has more than 400 feet (122 m) of elevation and there is no defined trail. As you climb (you will use your hands), you'll have incredible views of the other rocks in the canyon. The spire is an almost vertical climb. You can walk around Bell Rock.

Second, near downtown is Airport Mesa, which requires three miles (4.8 km) of hiking to get to the top, although you can also park near the top and climb down.

Third is Cathedral Rock, which rises two miles (3.2 km) straight uphill. It has a specific spot that is thought to be its own energy vortex. There is a hiking trail, but in order to truly climb it, you need experience.

Finally, you might want to visit Boynton Canyon vortex. There are famous caves and trails here that allow you to walk through the red rocks. Its specific vortex site is called Kachina Woman.

Not everyone has the same experience of these energy vortexes. Some people feel the energy spirals downward into the ground, while others feel it enlivens them, inspiring creativity and happiness.

To make sure no aspect of Sedona's magic landscape would be interrupted, the town became a certified International Dark Sky Community in 2014. This means that business and townspeople need to abide by specific guidelines to make sure artificial light will not disturb the view of stars.

Sedona and its people are deeply connected and respectful to the landscape, which includes the sky. If you have never seen a sky full of stars, it's difficult to explain just what you are missing because of the way light pollution disrupts the night sky.

People sometimes use the term *magic* to refer to the feeling that permeates those who visit in Sedona, but it could just be that people aren't used to locations that are so wide open and natural.

To that end, its important, if you visit Sedona, to be quiet. That doesn't mean not talking or sharing moments with friends and family. Instead, it means being open and receptive to the energy of the earth. Conversation can disrupt your receptivity to what the earth offers. There are, of course, numerous YouTube videos of "experts" describing what you should feel at an energy vortex, but the real point is to connect to the earth and that means remaining silent and using your senses to experience the world.

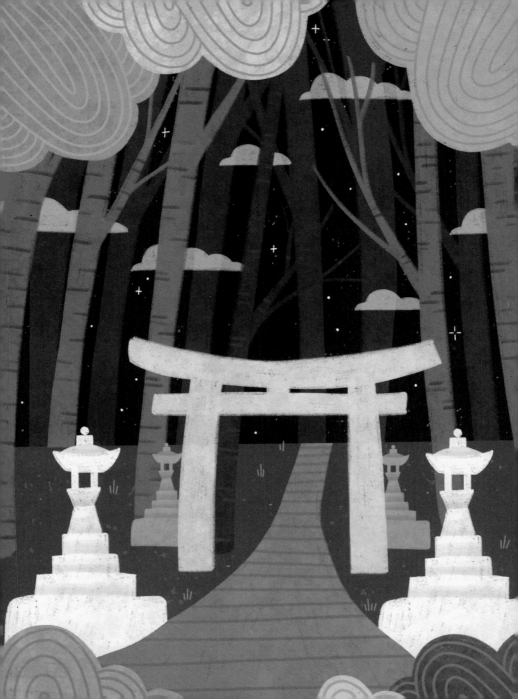

Japanese Forests

In the 1980s, Japanese scientists and doctors began to quantify a common practice among those who lived in or near forests: *shinrin-yoku*, which means "forest bathing." It isn't just the ground that connects us to the earth when we're in forests. The trees, fresh air, sounds of nature, and sense of quiet help create not just calm, but better health. In fact, ecotherapy, or nature therapy, is the practice of spending time in nature to benefit both physical and mental health. Researchers have found that two hours a week seem to make a positive difference, and that doesn't have to be all at once; daily walks are just as beneficial.

Japan has numerous locations that the country has named "Forest Therapy Roads," which are walking paths that have been scientifically evaluated and judged to be physiologically and psychologically beneficial. Forest Therapy Roads are leisurely walking environments with gentle slopes and wide paths. Forest bathing isn't hiking or strenuous walking.

One of Japan's great forests is Aokigahara Forest, which has views of Mt. Fuji. Another, Akasawa Natural Recreational Forest, is a coniferous forest. Another magical location is the Bamboo Forest Trail in Kyoto. Consider visiting the Shirakami Mountains, a World Natural Heritage site. The Kii Peninsula is home to Yoshino-Kumano National Park, which includes a Japanese beech tree forest. Finally, Yakushima National Park has a unique ecosystem that is home to 1,900 flora species and subspecies and 150 bird species. It is home to a primeval forest composed of cedar trees called yakusugi, which are more than a thousand years old.

FOREST BATHING

Although it's okay to bring your phone, just in case you'll need it, if you can, turn it off and put it away for your time in the forest. Try to walk without speaking, even if you are with a friend.

Rely on your senses for this experience. Touch: feel free to gently touch the trees. Smell: breathe in their scent. Sound: listen to the breeze and the animals. Sight: look closely at the leaves and the ground. You probably won't taste anything, but if it's raining, open your mouth and let the water in!

Black Hills, South Dakota

With its unfortunate political and economic history, the Black Hills are worthy of their own book (like many of the other locations with a connection to grounding), but you can consider visiting this area in the northern United States to ground yourself in the landscape, not its history of greed and racism (Mount Rushmore was built on a site sacred to the Sioux, and its carving was done by a member of the Ku Klux Klan).

Of course, the Black Hills were a beautiful landscape long before they were "discovered" by miners who overran the place looking for gold. That's because, like many locations around the world, the hills are filled with minerals, including quartz, copper, silver, lead, mica, and feldspar. Before Americans began to mine the Black Hills, the federal government signed a treaty in 1868 setting the area aside as part of the Great Sioux Reservation. Once miners discovered gold, Americans stole back the land in 1877. It is still under legal dispute between the U.S. government and the Sioux.

There are many walking and hiking trails in this area, from gentle slopes to intense climbing. Many of them are found in Custer State Park, which is unfortunate, as it was named for the general whose racist "last stand" was nearby. Underneath all that history, of course, is the earth, and for our purposes, the history begins and ends with the land. According to the U.S. Forest Service, the Black Hills look very much liked they did 40 million years ago, and they are a wonderful place to ground yourself with a walking meditation.

WALKING MEDITATION

For this meditation, be mindful of everything around you; each time you notice something outside of your body, acknowledge it.

First, find a spot where you want to start. Stand facing one direction and take in everything you see. Do this by telling yourself what you see. For example, "I see trees. I see a mountain. I see the sky." Be as specific as you can and, when you feel ready, make a quarter turn and do the same thing. Do this four times, facing in four directions.

Now, begin to walk, still "talking" to yourself (you don't have to do this aloud). Notice not only what you see, but also how your feet feel taking each step. If you feel overwhelmed by all you notice, stop and take some deep breaths. Remember not to judge yourself or what you're seeing. When that happens, simply stand still and go back to noticing. Notice without judgment or commentary.

At some point, your grounding should feel like you forget yourself and you feel one with the landscape. Compare this type of walk with the type of walk you normally take in which you may get lost in your thoughts and not even notice the details of everything around you.

When you are ready, find another spot to end your walk and repeat what you did in the beginning, turning in all four directions to notice everything around you.

Practicing this type of awareness is very helpful for relieving the habit of "multitasking." According to the *Journal of Experimental Psychology: Human Perception and Performance*, multitasking is less efficient than trying to focus on one activity at a time. There is an exception, though; it's likely you have noticed that you are most creative when you are walking, showering, or doing something like the dishes. Why is that? According to an article in *Psychology of Aesthetics, Creativity, and the Arts,* when we let our mind wander, we are at our most creative.

Therefore, don't be surprised if, because you are focused on the landscape and your mind is wandering from worries and concerns, you suddenly have an unexpected idea or a solution to a problem. Bring a notebook and pencil. Write that idea down! Don't judge yourself for thinking and not noticing the landscape. This is one of the benefits of walking meditations.

Bath, England

A UNESCO World Heritage Site, Bath is named for its water. It is one of the great spa towns with hot springs, and its baths were constructed in a public square in 70 CE. For many hundreds of years, visitors have believed its waters have healing powers. You can still bathe in the Roman baths. The warm, mineral-rich waters come from deep underground, and more than a million liters of steaming spring water fills the baths every day. Hot spring bathing is a public endeavor with guests wearing bathing suits. For private bathing, a number of hotels and resorts in the area have rooms in which you can bathe by yourself.

BATHS

People have long recognized the healing power of a good soak in the tub. You can enhance the experience with dim lighting, candles, soft music, and aromatherapy. Adding a sachet of dried herbs, such as lavender, rose, and chamomile, is soothing to the skin and the nervous system. Don't stay in too long—fifteen minutes is a good amount of time—or the hot water will dry out your skin. Extend the grounding experience by getting into a fluffy robe and moisturizing your skin with a soothing lotion.

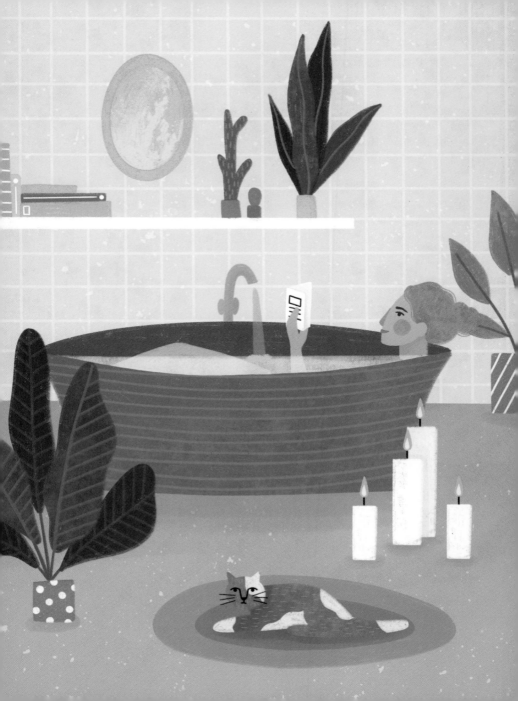

Bear Lake, Romania

There are many saltwater lakes in the world—in Utah, Israel/Jordan, and Romania. In these places, you can effortlessly float in the water. As you probably know, some of these lakes are so salty that they are "dead," as in the Dead Sea, because their salinity is so high, little-to-no life exists.

Despite this, salt water is good for people. In fact, it is especially good for reducing pain and seems to ease autoimmune symptoms, according to the National Ingredients Resource Center. Salt bathing helps with poison ivy and wound healing. Also, natural mineral salts restore the skin's mineral balance.

One of Romania's salt lakes, Bear Lake, is the result of a heliothermic (sun plus heat) phenomenon, which allows the lake to reach 95°F (35°C). Bear Lake is so interesting because fresh water from two nearby brooks flows into the lake and forms a very thin layer on top of the salt water. The sun hits the fresh water and warms up the salt water underneath, while the fresh water also insulates the salt water, so it doesn't rise to the surface.

To keep this natural system from being overly disrupted by humans, bathing is limited in Bear Lake. In fact, humans and climate change have disrupted many of the great salt lakes around the world. Fortunately, you can swim in saltwater pools, and you can also relax in a salt bath.

SALT BATHS

It's impossible to recreate a true saltwater bath, but you can do the next best thing and soak in Epsom salts. Epsom salts are not actually salt but magnesium sulfate. However, like salt, they dissolve in water and the mixture is grounding. Research has shown that Epsom salts can help ease muscle aches by rebalancing the mineral levels in your body, including electrolytes, which is why so many athletes soak in Epsom salts.

An Epsom salt bath doesn't require anything more than running warm water, pouring Epsom salts, which are sold under a number of brand names, into the water, and getting into the tub. A 2023 study published in the *International Journal of Health Sciences and Research* found that Epsom salts were effective in reducing the pain associated with arthritis.

You shouldn't use Epsom salts in a tub with jets. Instead, pour the salts under warm to hot running water and then, once they have dissolved, enjoy a soak for up to fifteen minutes. Don't keep adding more water, because too much time in the tub and the salts is drying to the skin.

When you get out of the tub, pat your skin until it's a little damp, not wet. Then, cover your body in a lotion made from natural ingredients, such as shea butter. This creates a barrier that prevents the water from evaporating from your skin. Cover up with socks and pajamas to remain comfortable once you leave the warm bathroom. Consider covering your head, too, until you acclimate to the temperature in your home.

Great Blue Hole, Belize

If you have ever wondered whether any oceans are deep enough to go to the center of the earth, you might feel inspired by the Great Blue Hole, just off the coast of Belize. No, it's not as deep as the center of the earth, but it sure looks like it is! The great oceanographer Jacques Cousteau called it one of the greatest scuba diving spots on the planet.

Maybe you're wondering how a place so deep could be considered "grounding," but seeing such a beautiful and inspirational place is spiritually grounding. The Great Blue Hole is also an experience "of earth." Remember, earth is made up of 71 percent water.

The Great Blue Hole is a circular marine sinkhole. It is just over 1,000 feet (305 m) across and just over 400 feet (122 m) deep. It is part of the Belize Barrier Reef Reserve System, which is a UNESCO World Heritage Site. The hole has caves on its floor (yes, submarines have descended to its floor).

Scuba divers still love to explore the Great Blue Hole, because it has numerous fish, including parrotfish and reef sharks. Remember, even when you are snorkeling or scuba diving, there is ground underneath you (sand) and to the side of you (coral reef). We truly only leave the ground when we fly.

If you can't get to the Great Blue Hole, simply keep an image of it in your mind's eye. Or you can float in the ocean or a lake while you do this meditation. A pool, a bath, or a footbath is also an option.

WATER MEDITATION

If you can, get a small water fountain that allows you to hear the sound of water flowing and bubbling. Another option is to turn on a rainfall or waterfall recording or video to listen to the sound of water flowing.

Spend a few minutes considering your interpretation of water's symbolism. Do you see it as something that flows continuously without blockages? Do you see it as something adaptable, able to change direction easily when necessary? Water's meaning to you is private. There is no right or wrong way to think about it.

Sit or lie down in a comfortable position. Take some time to inhale deeply and, when you exhale, consciously focus on relaxing one muscle or area of your body at a time. Notice where you feel some tension and focus on that body part. Do this for as long as you need to until you start to feel as if your body doesn't have edges, as if you're one with the water.

Move your consciousness away from your body and bring to mind a problem that has been bothering you. Imagine it as a box with hard sides and edges. Now, think of yourself as a body of water; instead of being stopped by the box or having to go through it, you are able to move around it. The box doesn't change, but it also doesn't get in your way. Instead, you remain whole, but you still move around the box. Keep inhaling and exhaling slowly while you take your time moving around the box.

Eventually, notice that you are past the box. The box is the same, but you have moved past it. Continue breathing deeply until you feel that the box no longer matters, that it is okay for the box to be a box—you don't have to change it or bring it along with you on your journey.

When you're ready, acknowledge that you, as a body of water, are still whole and the box is no longer in your way or with you on your journey. You have left it behind and are moving forward with your life.

GROUNDING
FOODS

———

"Let food by thy medicine and medicine be thy food."

HIPPOCRATES

M ichael Pollan, author of *Food Rules*, gives the easiest and best advice when it comes to eating: "Eat food, not too much, and mostly plants." Isn't everything we eat "food"? No. If it is made in a factory, it's not food. It's a product designed for eating, but it's rarely nutritious or healthy.

A potato, for example, has fiber and nutrients. It is relatively low in calories on its own. Potato chips, on the other hand, are high in calories, have added fats and salt, and contain no nutrients. When we eat a small potato (remember the second rule, "not too much") and top it with a bit of sour cream (a fermented food, which we will discuss later), we are eating real food.

One of the most important aspects of grounding foods is eating with the seasons. For generations, before Clarence Birdseye invented freezing and transporting foods, changing diets throughout the year was part of farming and living "close to the ground." Now, fresh foods are available to most of us throughout the year, so we eat strawberries, typically a summer fruit, in winter and oranges, a winter fruit, in summer.

Eating for the season is one aspect of Ayurvedic principles. Ayurveda is an alternative system of medicine with roots in India. It has not been widely studied by Western science, but many of its basic tenets, including eating with the seasons, have been adopted by people in the West.

Ayurvedic experts believe that every food has a unique energy and affects our bodies in a specific manner. This makes perfect sense, of course. Apples are high in fiber, vitamin C, and potassium, while pineapples have vitamin B6, copper, and niacin. The truth is, both fruits share many nutrients, but the point is that when Western medical professionals talk about eating a "balanced diet," they are referring to the same qualities of food to which Ayurvedic experts refer.

Western medicine has found that food is healing, and those beliefs are shared by many cultures: Chicken soup is Jewish penicillin, an apple a day keeps the doctor away, the Japanese offer miso soup to sick people, and borscht, a Russian staple, may help lower blood pressure.

In this chapter, we'll explore five types of foods that are grounding, offer some tips on how to cook with them, and give you some easy recipes to get started.

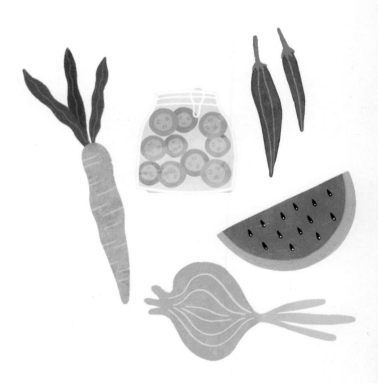

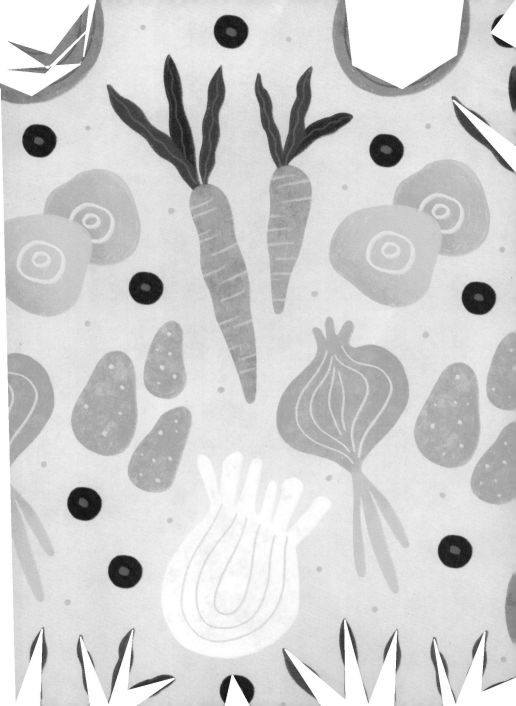

ROOT VEGETABLES

Not surprisingly, root vegetables, which, of course, grow in the ground (thus the name *root*), are an ideal nutrition source. Full of vitamins and minerals, as well as fiber, they are a great food group around which to plan your meals. You can ground yourself with these foods at every meal. Root vegetables include carrots, onions, potatoes, celery root, kohlrabi, parsnips, rutabagas, radishes, turnips, onions, and beets. These foods are easy to grow, so they make great additions to your garden. Root vegetables range through all the colors of the rainbow and "eating the rainbow" is another good food rule to follow.

According to the National Institutes of Health, the nutritional benefits of root vegetables include helping to regulate metabolic health, such as glucose and lipid levels, as well as blood pressure. Root vegetables also include many antioxidants and have prebiotic and anticancer properties. Antioxidants are vitamins, minerals, and other compounds in foods that neutralize free radicals, which contribute to aging and poor health. When we eat these nutrients, versus taking them as supplements, they are more beneficial to our health.

Many root vegetables can be eaten raw, but they can also be roasted, baked, steamed, sautéed, or pickled.

ROASTED VEGETABLES WITH QUINOA

YIELD: 4 SERVINGS

½ butternut squash, peeled and diced

20 Brussels sprouts, trimmed and halved

¼ cup (60 ml) olive oil

Salt and pepper

1 teaspoon paprika

¾ cup plus 2 tablespoons (177 ml plus 30 ml) water

½ cup (86 g) white quinoa

1 garlic clove

2 tablespoons (32 g) tahini

3 tablespoons (45 ml) apple cider vinegar

¼ cup (12 g) fresh chives, minced

¼ cup (24 g) flat leaf parsley,

¼ cup (24 g) cilantro, minced (optional)

2½ cups (203 g) baby spinach

This is a fantastic fall dish, but the tahini gives it a kick that makes it feel fresh and spring-like. If you're not familiar with tahini, it's something that should be in your fridge, as it can be mixed with chickpeas for homemade hummus and added to sour cream for a dip. Tahini is a sesame seed paste that is nutritious and rich in antioxidants. Likewise, apple cider vinegar has been shown to have many health benefits, including being antimicrobial and full of antioxidants. Of course, the vegetables are full of fiber, vitamins, and minerals, and the quinoa has healthy protein. You can store this in the fridge for a few days and eat it for lunch during the week.

1 Preheat oven to 425°F (220°C). Put squash and Brussels sprouts on baking sheet. Toss with 2 tablespoons (30 ml) oil, and season with salt and paprika. Roast for 25 to 30 minutes, stirring when halfway done to cook evenly.

2 As that cooks, bring ¾ cup (177 ml) water to a boil. Add quinoa and a pinch of salt. Reduce heat to low, cover, and simmer. The water should be absorbed after 15 minutes. Fluff with a fork. Transfer to a bowl.

3 In a food processor, pulse garlic, tahini, vinegar, remaining water, chives, parsley, and cilantro if you are using it. Add salt and pepper to taste.

4 Rinse the spinach well, because you are going to serve it raw.

5 In a large bowl, mix tahini mixture with quinoa and vegetables. Add spinach. Season with salt and pepper to taste. Serve.

VEGETABLE COBBLER

This is a very adaptable recipe. You can put the vegetable mixture in a premade pie shell and make pot pie (this is a cobbler because it doesn't have a bottom crust; with both crusts it is a pot pie). You can also vary the mixture and use whatever fall or winter vegetables you have on hand. It's a terrific recipe for vegetables that are getting old. Filled with fiber and lots of nutrients, the healthiness quotient is kicked up by adding buckwheat flour to the dough.

YIELD: 6 SERVINGS

1 cup (240 ml) vegetable broth

1 tablespoon (8 g) cornstarch

1 parsnip, peeled and cut into bite-sized pieces

1 russet potato, peeled and diced

1 celery root, peeled and diced

1 yellow onion, chopped into bite-sized pieces

3 carrots, peeled and diced

½ cup (48 g) minced fresh parsley

1 teaspoon salt

Pepper to taste

4 tablespoons (56 g) butter, cut into small pieces

FOR THE DOUGH

1 cup (120 g) all-purpose flour

½ cup (60 g) buckwheat flour

1 tablespoon (14 g) baking powder

1 teaspoon salt

6 tablespoons (84 g) cold butter, cut into small pieces

¾ cup (180 ml) heavy cream

Extra flour to roll out the dough

1   Preheat the oven to 325°F (170°C).

2   In a small bowl, combine the cornstarch and the vegetable broth.

3   Put all the vegetables in a 13-inch x 9-inch (33 cm × 23 cm) glass baking dish. Pour the vegetable broth mixture over the vegetables and stir. Add salt and pepper to taste. Dot bits of butter over the vegetables.

4   Now, make the dough: Mix the flours, baking powder, and salt in a large mixing bowl.

5   Put the pieces of butter in the dough and, using your fingers, crumble the butter into the flour mixture until it resembles coarse sand.

6   Slowly pour the cream into the flour mixture, stirring with a fork.

7   Begin to form the dough into a ball.

8   On a floured surface, roll the dough to ¼ inch (6 mm) thick until it is slightly larger than the baking dish.

9   Place the dough in the baking dish and use a fork to poke holes across the surface.

10   Bake in the preheated oven for 30 minutes, or until the dough is fully browned and the vegetables bubbling hot when you serve.

WHITE BEAN, KALE, AND LEEK SOUP

YIELD: 6 SERVINGS

¼ cup (60 ml) vegetable oil

8 ounces (227 g) mushrooms, cleaned and chopped

3 leeks, cleaned and thinly sliced thin (white and light green parts)

3 carrots, cut into ½-inch (1.3 cm) pieces

1 bunch kale, stemmed and shredded into 2-inch (5 cm) pieces

15 ounces (420 g) white beans

1 quart (960 ml) vegetable stock

Salt and pepper

Chopped fresh parsley (optional)

This recipe is grounding for a few reasons. First, it contains more than a few "from the earth" ingredients, including white beans, leeks, carrots, mushrooms, and kale. Second, because it is warm and hearty, but not high in calories, it is nourishing but not heavy.

1   Heat the oil in a stockpot over medium heat.

2   Add the mushrooms, leeks, and carrots, and cook, stirring frequently, until slightly softened.

3   Add the kale and cook, stirring frequently, until soft and wilted.

4   Add the beans and stock and stir to combine. Cook for 15 minutes.

5   Add salt and pepper to taste. Sprinkle each serving with fresh parsley, if desired. Serve.

PARSNIP SOUP
WITH WALNUTS

Adapted from Marcus Off Duty *by Marcus Samuelsson. Samuelsson's original recipe calls for Indian spices, which are warming, and a lot of garlic. This version is milder and brings out the sweetness of the pears.*

YIELD: 6 SERVINGS

2 tablespoons (30 ml) extra-virgin olive oil

2½ pounds (1.1 kg) parsnips, peeled and chopped

1 teaspoon kosher salt, plus more for seasoning

2 teaspoons (5 g) cardamom

4 cups (944 ml) water

3 cups (708 ml) vegetable broth

1½ cups (354 ml) heavy cream

Ground black pepper, to taste

FOR THE TOPPING

1 teaspoon extra-virgin olive oil

½ cup (60 g) walnuts, chopped

1 tablespoon (15 ml) fresh lemon juice

1½ teaspoons walnut oil

1 small Bosc or d'Anjou pear, finely chopped

1 tablespoon (4 g) chopped parsley

1 tablespoon (4 g) chopped tarragon

Kosher salt, to taste

Ground black pepper, to taste

1 Heat the olive oil in a large saucepan over medium heat.

2 Add the parsnips to the saucepan, stirring until light brown, about 5 minutes.

3 Stir in the cardamom and 1 teaspoon of salt. Continue stirring for 2 minutes.

4 Add the water, vegetable broth, and cream, and bring to a simmer. Cook until the vegetables are soft, about 25 minutes.

5 Remove from the heat and, with an immersion blender, puree until very smooth.

6 To make the topping, place a medium skillet over low heat. Add the olive oil and heat. Stir in the walnuts and toast, stirring, until golden, about 3 minutes. Remove from the heat and add the lemon juice. Scrape the mixture into a small bowl and toss with the walnut oil. Cool to room temperature, then stir in the pear, parsley, and tarragon. Season with salt and pepper to taste.

7 Pour the soup into a clean saucepan and add lemon juice. Stir, then season with salt and pepper.

8 Divide the soup among several bowls and then sprinkle the topping over each one.

FERMENTED FOODS

For generations, fermented foods were considered helpful because they extended the shelf life of fresh foods, turning cucumbers into pickles and cabbage into sauerkraut. Recently, though, nutrition research has found that fermented foods have many health benefits. The microorganisms that instigate the fermentation process synthesize vitamins and minerals, create helpful enzymes that facilitate digestion, and remove non-nutrients during the process. Biologically active peptides, compounds produced by the fermentation bacteria, also have health benefits. One of these is conjugated linoleic acids (CLA), which help lower blood pressure. Others have prebiotic and antimicrobial properties, making them good for the digestive system.

You can pickle foods quickly by cooking them in boiling water combined with salt, sugar, spices, and herbs. It's fun to experiment with vegetables and the other ingredients, including different types of vinegar, to get flavors you like.

Not all fermented foods are pickled. Yogurt, sour cream, and other dairy products are fermented with live bacteria cultures. Like pickles, yogurt and sour cream are one food, milk or cream, turned into another with the use of an added ingredient.

Although fermentation processes differ, all fermentation creates medicinal value. According to the National Institutes of Health, yogurt has calcium; numerous minerals, including potassium and phosphorus; and vitamins A, B_2, and B_{12}. I1t is nutrient dense, but low in calories, if you don't add a lot of sugar, which store-bought yogurt often has. To keep yogurt nutritious, buy plain yogurt and add a teaspoon of honey or fresh fruit (or both!), which allows you to control both the flavor and the calories.

According to a 2022 article in *ReNew: Technology for a Sustainable Future*, fermentation is a way to ground to the planet, as it encourages us to keep food from one season to use in another season. For example, we grow many vegetables in summer, but to use them in winter we need to preserve them, and fermenting that produce is an ancient way to do this.

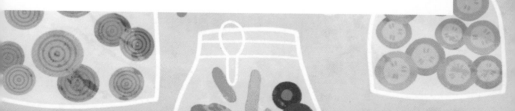

SZECHUAN BRAISED BEAN CURD WITH VEGETABLES

YIELD: 4 SERVINGS

6 to 8 tablespoons (90 to 129 ml) oil

1 pound (455 g) tofu, cubed and dried

1 small eggplant, peeled and cut into strips

3 cups (690 g) sliced mushrooms

2 cups (166 g) green beans, diced

¼ cup plus 3 tablespoons (60 ml plus 45 ml) water

1 tablespoon (15 g) chili paste

2 cloves garlic

3 tablespoons (54 g) tamari

4½ tablespoons (68 ml) rice wine or dry sherry

This dish is categorized under fermented because tamari is fermented, although tofu is not. If you have a wok, you can use that. Either way, try to make sure your pan is hot, but the oil should not smoke.

1 In a wok or skillet over medium-high heat, warm about 3 tablespoons (45 ml) oil.

2 When the oil is hot, add half the tofu and stir-fry. One golden, move the tofu to a paper towel–lined plate. Wipe down the pan, then add more oil, and repeat with the rest of the tofu.

3 Add the remaining oil to the pan and, once hot, add the eggplant and fry for 3 minutes, stirring the whole time.

4 Add the mushrooms, green beans, and garlic. Keep stirring. If you need to, add more oil.

5 Add ¼ cup (60 ml) water. Cover the pan and let steam for 5 minutes.

6 In a small bowl, mix the chili paste, tamari, rice wine, and 3 tablespoons (45 ml) water.

7 Lower the heat to medium and add the tofu back to the pan, along with the tamari mixture. Stir until hot, about 3 minutes.

8 Divide the mixture over 4 bowls and serve.

HOMEMADE PICKLES

Truly one of the greatest treats, pickles began as a method to keep summer vegetables for winter. Cucumbers are the obvious one, but you can pickle so many other vegetables, such as onions. Because you aren't boiling or sealing Mason jars, these pickles will not keep through winter. You have to eat them within a few days, and that's one reason this recipe isn't for a large batch. Instead, you're making a small amount to use in salads or on sandwiches. Kirby cucumbers are best; avoid long English cucumbers.

YIELD: 8 SERVINGS

¼ cup (70 g) kosher salt

¾ cup (180 ml) boiling water

3 ice cubes

1½ pounds (680 g) cucumbers, thinly sliced

3 cloves garlic, crushed

1 small bunch fresh dill or 1 tablespoon (2 g) dried dill

1   In a large bowl, combine the salt and boiling water. Stir to dissolve the salt and then add the ice cubes. Let cool to room temperature.

2   Add the cucumbers, garlic, and dill. Cover with cold water.

3   Put a plate in the bowl with something heavy on top to keep the pickles in the water. They should be immersed, not squished.

4   Taste the pickles anywhere from 8 to 12 hours later to see if they taste the way you want.

5   Refrigerate them in the brine in Mason jars. They won't continue to pickle much more in the fridge.

NOTE: Cooks who turn cucumbers into pickles rarely use exact measurements. The amounts of water, garlic, salt, and dill (you can also use coriander and celery salt) are really to taste. This is another good reason to make small batches. Keep note of the flavors and amounts you like. The water amounts aren't that important, but you don't want the flavor to be too watered down. You can use the pickle brine in cocktails or to cook other foods.

EGGPLANT IN YOGURT

This recipe is based on an Afghan dish, borani banjan. *Typically served as an appetizer or side dish, the eggplant is usually fried in oil, but here it is cooked in an air fryer, making the preparation easier. If you shop in Middle Eastern stores, you can likely find the Kashmiri spices that Afghan cooks use. This recipe calls for chili powder, but you can experiment with other powdered spices and peppers.*

YIELD: 4 SERVINGS

1½ cups (225 g) full-fat Greek yogurt

2 garlic cloves, grated

3 teaspoons (17 g) salt, divided

1 teaspoon chili powder, divided

4 tablespoons (60 ml) water, divided

4 Japanese eggplants, cut into 1-inch (2.5 cm) slices

¼ cup (60 ml) vegetable oil

6 plum tomatoes, chopped

3 tablespoons (26 g) pomegranate seeds

8 mint leaves

1   In a medium mixing bowl, combine the yogurt, garlic, 1 teaspoon salt, ¼ teaspoon chili powder, and 2 tablespoons (30 ml) water. Cover and put in the refrigerator.

2   Heat the air fryer to 400°F (200°C).

3   In a large mixing bowl, combine the eggplant, vegetable oil, 1 teaspoon salt, and ½ teaspoon chili powder.

4   Once the air fryer is up to temperature, place the eggplant in the basket and cook for 12 minutes, or until the eggplant is easy to pierce with a fork.

5   In a cast-iron pan over medium-high heat, add the tomatoes, 1 teaspoon salt, 2 tablespoons (30 ml) water, and remaining chili powder. Cook for 5 minutes, or until the tomatoes start to break down into a sauce.

6   Let all of the components, except the yogurt, come to room temperature.

7   Spread the yogurt across the bottom of a large shallow dish. Top with the eggplant slices in a single layer. Spread the tomato mixture over the eggplant. Sprinkle pomegranate seeds and mint on top, and then serve.

YOGURT SMOOTHIE

This smoothie recipe can be varied with any types of berries. Instead of beets, substitute kale or spinach to make a green smoothie. Keep the fruit in, though, to make the smoothie sweet and not bitter. Feel free to add seeds, too, including chia or flax.

This is a simple recipe, and you can change it up to include your favorite fruits, juices, vegetables, and sweeteners.

YIELD: 1 SERVING

⅓ cup (80 g) plain yogurt

¼ cup (60 ml) orange juice

¾ cup (112 g) frozen berries (any kind)

¼ cup (40 g) diced beets, raw or roasted

1 teaspoon honey

Ice cubes or water

1   Place all the ingredients in a blender and blend for 1 minute, until smooth. Serve immediately.

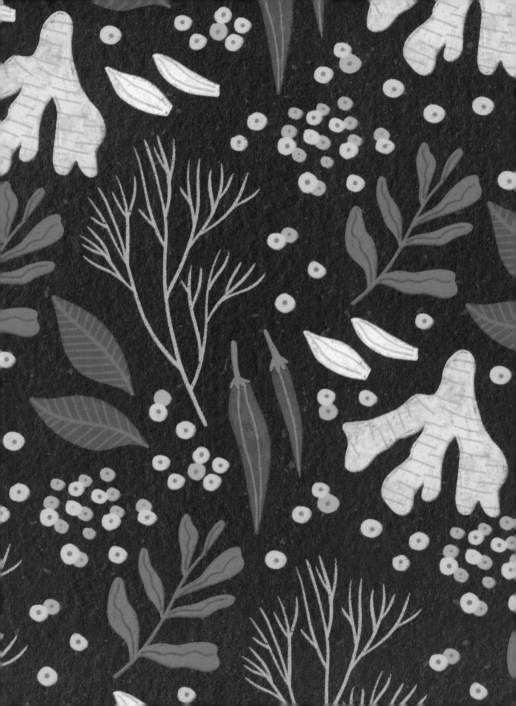

SPICES AND HERBS

The warmth of cinnamon. The freshness of parsley. The comfort of ginger. The bite of basil. Not only do spices and herbs add flavor and vitality to a dish, but researchers have found they have medicinal benefits as well. So, not only do they move a meal from good to great, but they are good—great—for us, too.

Spices come from a variety of plant parts, including bark, flowers, fruits, leaves, rhizomes, seeds, and stems. They are not green, typically, unlike herbs, and generally come from non-woody plants. Herbs come from the green leafy parts and young, tender stems. Some foods that we consider spice, such as chile peppers, are actually fruit, and it's the dried seeds that we use as spice. You can buy spices whole or ground, and herbs are available fresh or dried. One of the best ways to add spice to your dishes is through blends, and many cultures feature specific blends, such as curry, masala, and za'atar.

If you want to use less sugar when you cook, then experiment with spices, because their intense flavors make it easier to not need sweetness for flavor. Anise, for example, is thirteen times sweeter than table sugar, so adding it to recipes will allow you to cut down on sugar. It does taste like licorice, so it's not for everyone.

Many spices and herbs, such as ginger, mint, mustard, horseradish, and turmeric, have grounding medicinal properties. They are grounding because they come from nature—ginger is a rhizome (underground stem) of a tropical flowering plant. Mint and mustard can help clear the nasal passages.

Using herbs and spices brings plants and nature to our cooking, especially for dishes that may not be plant-centered, such as meats. Herbs bring a bright green brightness to dishes, much like the greens that you see in forests, while spices often come from parts of plants that you touch or that are below ground. It's important to remember that grounding is a sensory experience and when it comes to herbs and spices, that sense is taste, the one sense that you don't excite while when you walk in woods or bury your feet in the sand.

HIKING BARS

These are the perfect bars to take on a hike, because they stay solid and have enough sugar to give you energy. When you take a long hike, it's important to not only hydrate but also to refuel every 60 to 90 minutes so that you don't get tired.

YIELD: 18 BARS

6 tablespoons (84 g) butter

⅓ cup (64 g) sugar

⅓ cup (64 g) packed dark brown sugar

2 eggs

1½ cups (180 g) all-purpose flour

½ teaspoon salt

½ teaspoon baking powder

½ teaspoon cinnamon

¼ teaspoon ground cloves

¼ teaspoon ground ginger

2 tablespoons (42 g) dark molasses mixed with 1 tablespoon (15 ml) warm water

½ cup (80 g) raisins

½ cup (56 g) pecans, chopped

1   Preheat the oven to 350°F (177°C). Line 2 baking sheets with parchment paper, and then grease the parchment paper.

2   Place the butter and sugars in a medium mixing bowl. Cream using an electric mixer, and then add 1 egg.

3   In a separate bowl, mix the flour, salt, baking powder, cinnamon, cloves, and ginger.

4   Combine the two mixtures, and then stir in the molasses mixture.

5   Fold in the raisins and nuts.

6   Divide the dough in half and place each half in the middle of a cookie sheet. With floured hands, shape the dough into strips that are about 9 × 3 inches (22 × 8 cm).

7   In a small bowl, lightly beat the remaining egg. Use a pastry brush to brush the egg wash on the top of the dough.

8   Bake for 15 to 20 minutes, until the tops begin to brown. While the dough logs are still warm, slice into 9 bars. Let cool and serve.

CORN AND BUTTERMILK SALAD WITH HERBS

YIELD: 8 SERVINGS

1 cup (240 ml) buttermilk

¼ cup (60 ml) extra-virgin olive oil

½ cup (120 g) sour cream

5 tablespoons (24 g) chopped dill

2 tablespoons (12 g) minced shallot

1 teaspoon minced garlic

Lots of salt and white or black pepper

10 cups (1.5 kg) cooked fresh corn

3 small Kirby cucumbers, quartered lengthwise and thinly sliced

This is a great salad to bring to a picnic. You need to get about 5 ears of corn and cook them, then slice the corn off the ears to use in the salad. Also, the dressing is very much to taste. You might want more garlic or to experiment with different herbs.

1   In a large bowl, mix buttermilk, oil, sour cream, dill, shallot, and garlic. Add salt and pepper.

2   Add corn and cucumbers to dressing. Toss everything and taste, adjusting seasonings. Put in fridge so flavors blend.

3   Bring to room temperature and toss well to serve.

WARM CINNAMON MUESLI

Cinnamon comes from the inner bark of a tropical tree, and research has found that it is beneficial in controlling blood sugar. Muesli is the Swiss version of granola, and you can serve it cooked, either hot or cold, or raw. Muesli can be a snack or a filling morning meal.

This is a simple recipe, and you can mix and match most of the ingredients, adding more of what you like and leaving out the flavors you don't enjoy. Therefore, there are suggested substitutions for most of the ingredients.

YIELD: 8 SERVINGS

1 cup (120 g) walnuts (or almonds, pecans, or a mixture), finely chopped

1 tablespoon (15 ml) maple syrup or honey

2 teaspoons ground cinnamon

2 tablespoons (25 g) light brown sugar (optional)

3 cups (240 g) rolled oats (not quick or instant)

10 Medjool dates (or raisins, dried cranberries, dried figs, dried apple, dried apricots, prunes, or a mixture), finely chopped

1 teaspoon salt

1 Preheat the oven to 350°F (180°C).

2 In a small bowl, toss the walnuts in the maple syrup, then add the cinnamon and brown sugar (if using), and toss to coat.

3 Line a baking sheet with parchment paper and spread the nuts in a single layer. Bake for 5 to 7 minutes, until golden. Remove from the oven and let cool.

4 Meanwhile, in a large bowl, combine the oats, dates, and salt.

5 When the nuts are fully cool, add to the oats and stir to combine.

6 Store in an airtight container at room temperature. You can serve the muesli cooked in milk, mixed with cottage cheese, or just out of a bowl.

CARDAMOM CRÈME BRÛLÉE

YIELD: 4 SERVINGS

1 quart (960 ml) heavy cream

3 green cardamom pods, crushed

6 large egg yolks

1½ cups (300 g) sugar, plus 2 tablespoons (25 g), divided

¼ teaspoon kosher salt

Crème brûlée is typically thought of as a fancy dish, but it is easy to make. It is custard made of cream, sugar, egg yolks, and flavoring, often vanilla extract. The word brûlée *refers to the top being caramelized, and, to do that, you can use a small kitchen torch or your broiler. You can also eat it without the crunchy top if you prefer.*

This dish uses cardamom pods, which you can find in the spice/baking aisle of most grocery stores. Cardamom is used in both sweet and savory dishes. Research has found that it contains chemicals that can fight inflammation. You will need four ramekins or other small oven-safe bowls or cups.

1 Preheat the oven to 325°F (170°C).

2 Combine the heavy cream and cardamom pods in a saucepan over medium-low heat. Bring the cream to a simmer and let it simmer gently for 10 minutes to infuse the cream with the cardamom. Remove from the heat and let cool. Strain out the cardamom pods.

3 Meanwhile, in a bowl, whisk together the egg yolks and 1½ cups (300 g) of the sugar until they are light in color and fully mixed (this will take a few minutes).

4 Whisk one-quarter of the cream into the eggs and sugar to temper the mixture. This prevents the eggs from curdling. Then, pour the egg/sugar mixture into the cream and whisk.

5 Pour the mixture into four 6-ounce (170 g) ramekins. Place the ramekins in a baking dish with high sides and fill the dish with boiling water to come halfway up the sides of the ramekins. Or you can put the ramekins in the baking dish, put the dish in the oven, then pour boiling water into the dish.

6 Bake for 45 minutes. Check toward the end, as the centers should jiggle. Don't overcook.

7 Remove the baking dish from the oven, remove the ramekins from the baking dish, and put the ramekins in the fridge until completely cool, about 5 hours.

8 Sprinkle the remaining 2 tablespoons (25 g) of sugar on top of each ramekin and, using a torch, caramelize the tops. If you don't have a torch or are uncomfortable using one, you can place the ramekins under the broiler for a few minutes, watching them carefully. Serve.

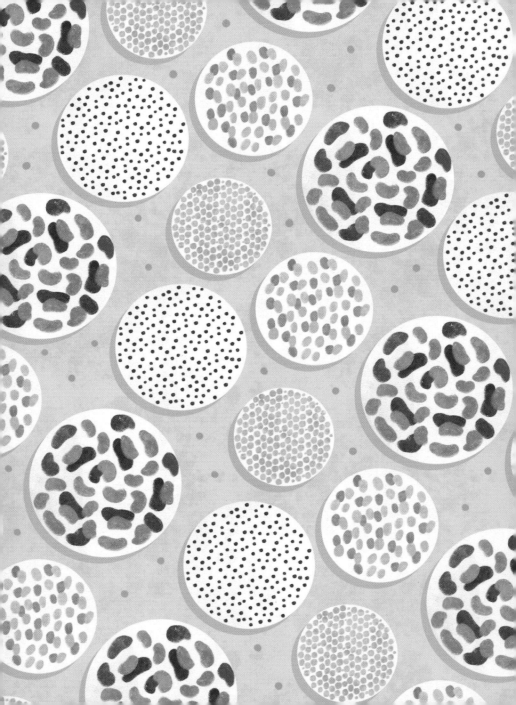

LEGUMES, BEANS, AND PULSES

You probably know that peas aren't nuts, but did you know that peanuts aren't either? Legumes are plants in the Fabaceae family, which includes lentils, broad beans, chickpeas, soybeans, lima beans, and peanuts. Their seeds are sometimes called "pulses." For example, a pea is the pulse of a peapod, which is a legume.

These foods are truly "of the earth." The soil feeds the legumes with nitrogen and, in exchange, the plant offers carbohydrates to bacteria in the soil. This is why farmers often use legume cover crops, such as soybeans, to "fix" nitrogen in the soil. When you eat these foods, you are not just eating the bean or pea, but the soil in which it grew.

Legumes, beans, and pulses are great sources of plant protein, folate, fiber, iron, and fatty acids. They also have a low glycemic index, which means they won't raise your blood sugar too much and are great foods for those with insulin sensitivity or diabetes. They are filling because of their high fiber content, too.

LENTIL BURGERS WITH LETTUCE AND YOGURT

YIELD: 4 SERVINGS

¾ cup (135 g) brown lentils, rinsed

3 cups (720 ml) water

Salt, to taste

1 shallot, minced

2 large eggs

1 cup (136 g) panko breadcrumbs, unflavored

2 tablespoons (20 g) parsley, minced

2 tablespoons (30 ml) olive oil

½ cup (75 g) Greek yogurt

Pinch cayenne pepper

1 head butter lettuce

Pickled onions

Lentils are extremely nutritious and high in protein, a perfect legume. They are notoriously difficult to cook properly, but you can't get canned lentils like you can get canned beans. However, fortunately, you can get cooked shelf-stable lentils in bags, usually in the international food grocery aisle. Sometimes these are already seasoned, and that's okay, as you can make the "burgers" with those flavors! This recipe includes instructions on how to cook the lentils from scratch.

1   Bring lentils and water to a boil in a small saucepan. Reduce to simmer, season with salt, and cook until tender, about 30 minutes. Drain and cool.

2   In a food processor, combine lentils, shallot, eggs, breadcrumbs, and parsley.

3   Heat olive oil in a skillet or non-stick pan, keep heat on medium. Using wet hands, shape ¼ cup (60 ml) of the lentil mixture into a patty and add to skillet. Make 4 patties. Cover skillet and cook for about 5 minutes on each side. When done, transfer to paper towel.

4   Meanwhile, add salt, cayenne, olive oil, and parsley to yogurt.

5   Place a lettuce leaf on plate, put one patty on each leaf, and top with yogurt mixture. Add pickled onions and serve.

CABBAGE ENCHILADAS

Usually made with tortillas, i.e., processed flour, and lots of meat, enchiladas may be delicious, but they aren't going to connect you to the Earth. That's why this variation substitutes cabbage for tortillas and beans for beef. It's lightened, too, by cutting down the cheese and pumping up the veggies. Remember that not everyone likes cilantro. You might want to play it safe and use parsley.

YIELD: 5 SERVINGS

10 green cabbage leaves

1 tablespoon (15 ml) olive oil

1 small onion, diced

1 small green pepper, diced

1 small red pepper, diced

1 carrot, peeled and diced

1 cup (113 g) broccoli rice

1 cup (113 g) cauliflower rice

2 cloves garlic

2 teaspoons (6 g) ground cumin

2 teaspoons (6 g) chili powder

2 cups (520 g) canned red beans

1½ cups (355 ml) red enchilada sauce

2 tablespoons (12 g) cilantro or parsley, minced

1½ cups (168 g) shredded Mexican cheese mixture

½ cup (124 g) sour cream

1 lime

1   Preheat oven to 350°F (177°C). Bring a large pot of water to a boil.

2   Using tongs, dip each cabbage leaf into the boiling water for about 30 seconds, and then transfer it to a paper towel–lined plate.

3   Heat oil in a large skillet over medium-high heat. Add onion, peppers, broccoli, cauliflower, and salt. Cook until softened.

4   Stir in the garlic, cumin, and chili powder, then add the beans, 1 cup (237 ml) enchilada sauce, and half the cilantro.

5   Remove the mixture from the heat, and put a giant spoonful on a cabbage leaf. Roll each leaf with the mixture like a burrito. Place in a 13 × 9-inch (33 × 23 cm) baking dish.

6   Spoon the rest of the enchilada sauce over the enchiladas and top with the cheese.

7   Place the baking dish in the preheated oven and bake for 20 minutes.

8   Combine the sour cream and lime juice.

9   Remove the baking dish from the oven and serve the enchiladas with a drizzle of sour cream mixture over the top. Garnish with cilantro.

LENTIL SALAD

This dish is based on a classic French recipe, which originally used lentils from Le Puy, a town in a French valley near the Loire River. It doesn't matter whether you use Puy lentils specifically. You can try the recipe with regular lentils that you get in your grocery store, or look for French green lentils from Bob's Red Mill and other online grocers.

This salad is not like an American salad in that it isn't lettuce-based, and it can be served warm. Also, it contains other grounding ingredients, including carrot, onion, and thyme. This salad is a perfect lunch, because it is filling and full of plant protein.

YIELD: 6 SERVINGS

1¼ cups (240 g) French green or regular lentils

3 fresh thyme sprigs

Salt and pepper

7 tablespoons (105 ml) olive oil, divided

1 carrot, peeled and finely diced

1 medium Vidalia onion, finely diced

1 tablespoon (15 ml) sherry vinegar

½ teaspoon Dijon mustard

1 small shallot, minced

Fresh parsley leaves

1   Rinse the lentils in a fine-mesh strainer and look through them, removing any that are discolored and any small stones.

2   Fill a large saucepan three-fourths of the way with water and add the lentils, thyme sprigs, and salt to taste. Bring the water to a boil, lower the heat, and simmer for 25 minutes, or until soft but not mushy. You may need to add more water. Remove from the heat and let lentils cool to room temperature.

3   Meanwhile, heat 3 tablespoons (45 ml) of the olive oil in a skillet over medium heat. Add the carrots and onions and season with salt and pepper. Cook, stirring, until tender, 6 to 8 minutes. Remove from the heat and set aside.

4   In a large bowl, mix the remaining 4 tablespoons (60 ml) of oil, vinegar, and mustard. Add salt and pepper to taste.

5   Remove thyme from the lentils, then add the lentils and vegetables to the bowl with the vinaigrette. Toss to coat and combine. Serve.

PEAS AND PEARL ONIONS

This is, admittedly, a simple dish. However, it is fantastic, grounding, and something that many people only make for the holiday table. That's so sad! If you ever crave something comforting with dinner, this is a good option. Ideally, get the peas straight from the pods (this is a good task for children to help with). Yes, it takes a long time to get all the peas you'll need, but that, too, is a grounding activity.

YIELD: 6 SERVINGS

1 cup (240 ml) whole milk, divided

1 whole clove

1 bay leaf

4 ounces (112 g) pearl or small onions

8 ounces (224 g) fresh peas

4 tablespoons (56 g) unsalted butter, divided

2 teaspoons salt, divided

1 tablespoon (8 g) all-purpose flour

1 teaspoon ground white pepper

¼ teaspoon nutmeg

Chopped fresh dill

½ cup (120 g) sour cream

1 Combine ¾ cup (180 ml) of the milk, clove, and bay leaf in a small saucepan over medium heat. Bring to a boil, and then decrease the heat to low. Simmer for 15 minutes. Strain into a medium bowl and discard the solids. Cover to keep warm.

2 Meanwhile, place the onions in a large skillet. Add enough water to immerse all the onions without covering them. Add 3 tablespoons (42 g) butter and 1 teaspoon salt. Cook over medium-high heat, stirring occasionally, until the liquid has evaporated and the onions are golden brown, about 12 minutes. Gently transfer the onions to a large plate.

3 Melt the remaining 1 tablespoon (14 g) butter in the same skillet over medium-low heat. Add the flour and whisk to combine. Continue to stir, picking up browned bits from the bottom of the pan, for 1 minute. Slowly whisk in the remaining ¼ cup (60 ml) milk and continue to cook, stirring, until thickened and bubbly, 3 to 4 minutes. Stir in the remaining 1 teaspoon salt, white pepper, and nutmeg. Stir in the peas and onions and heat through.

4 Top with sour cream and fresh dill and serve.

FRUITS

At the risk of being obvious, you know that fruit grows on trees or bushes and, thus, comes from the ground. Some fruits, of course, are closer to the ground than others. Whether grown on trees (apples, pineapples, grapefruit), bushes (strawberries, apricots), or vines (grapes), fruits are essentially a rainbow of good-for-you flavor, and each fruit brings different flavors and nutrients.

BAKED ACORN SQUASH

2 acorn squash, halved

4 tablespoons (56 g) salted butter

¼ cup (60 ml) maple syrup

Salt and pepper to taste

Like many foods, you likely consider squash a vegetable, but botanically it is in the fruit family. However you categorize it, acorn squash is a highly nutritious food. Like other orange foods, it is high in antioxidants, including vitamins C and A. Although this recipe calls for acorn squash, you can substitute other squashes. Not only that, but because it is a sweet recipe, you can serve it for dessert like a pudding if you are trying to eat less white flour and sugar. It is that delicious.

Speaking of its sweetness, real maple syrup is more nutritious than sugar. It is filled with healthy minerals, including manganese, zinc, calcium, potassium, magnesium, and a little iron.

1   Preheat oven to 400°F (200°C).

2   Line a baking sheet with parchment paper. Place the squash cut side down on the baking sheet and bake in the oven until you can easily stick a fork in them, about 45 minutes to 1 hour.

3   In a small saucepan over a low heat, melt the butter and maple syrup.

4   Remove the squash from the oven and scoop the flesh into a bowl. Mash until smooth.

5   Mix half the syrup into the squash, and transfer the squash to a serving bowl or spoon it out into small dishes. Pour a little syrup on top and serve.

FRUIT SALAD WITH CRÈME FRAÎCHE AND HONEY

You'll want to use fresh, preferably locally farm-grown fruit for this. Stick to the seasons for the freshest and most economical fruit.

Winter—apples, pears, citrus fruits, kiwi, grapes

Spring—apricots, kiwis, mangoes, cherries

Summer—strawberries, watermelon, peaches

Fall—apples, pears, persimmons, pomegranates

YIELD: 4 SERVINGS

4 cups (500 g) chopped fruits (any variety)

1 cup (240 g) crème fraîche or sour cream

¼ cup (80 g) honey

¼ cup (30 g) chopped nuts (any variety)

Fresh mint sprigs

1 Spoon a cup of chopped fruit into each of four bowls. Top the fruit with a dollop of crème fraîche. Drizzle a tablespoon of honey over the fruit and crème fraîche. Then, sprinkle the nuts over the fruit, crème fraîche, and honey. Add a sprig of mint on top.

NOTE: If you crave carbohydrate-rich treats at night, this is an excellent substitute for processed foods. All of the ingredients are natural and grounding, and a cup of fruit has 15 grams of carbs, the same amount as two Oreos. Of course, the honey has carbs, too (17 grams), but the crème fraîche and nuts add protein and fat, which slow the digestion of carbs, and you also get fiber with the fruit and nuts. All in all, this is a far more filling and nutritionally balanced choice than cookies or chips.

APPLE GALETTE

FOR THE CRUST

1 cup (120 g) buckwheat flour, plus more for rolling

½ cup (60 g) oat flour

2 teaspoons maple sugar

½ teaspoon salt

½ cup (112 g) unsalted butter, cold

5 tablespoons (75 ml) buttermilk, cold

FOR THE FILLING

1 tablespoon (8 g) oat flour

¼ teaspoon salt

½ cup (60 g) toasted pecans, chopped

4½ cups (500 g) very thinly sliced apples (peeled if desired)

3 tablespoons (36 g) firmly packed maple sugar

2 tablespoons (28 g) unsalted butter, cold, cubed

FOR THE TOPPING

1 large egg, beaten with 1 tablespoon (15 ml) water

Coarse sugar, for sprinkling

Although most desserts focus on sugar, you can find many more grounding recipes that feature fruits and even vegetables, which are naturally sweet and nutritious. Plus, because of their grounding qualities, they feel good to eat, not indulgent or "bad" for you. A galette is a free-form tart that has a rustic appearance.

This recipe features buckwheat flour, which is gluten-free, so this recipe is perfect to serve those who are sensitive to gluten. It has a nutty, earthy flavor and lots of good-for-you minerals, such as magnesium, manganese, phosphorus, potassium, copper, zinc, and iron. These are the types of nutrients that are processed out of white flour. Buckwheat flour also contains vitamins B_6, niacin, thiamin, and folate, as well as high-quality protein. The flour is actually ground, not processed. Sometimes, depending on the brand you buy, you will see bits of the ground hull in the flour. That just means more flavor. Don't worry, the apple taste will still shine through!

1 Preheat the oven to 400°F (200°C). Line a baking sheet with parchment paper.

2 To make the crust: In a medium bowl, combine the flours, maple sugar, and salt. Work in the cold butter until it's in pea-size chunks. Gradually stir in the buttermilk, using a fork. Start with 4 tablespoons (60 ml), adding more as needed to bring the dough together. Gather the dough into a ball, pat it into a disk ¾ inch (2 cm) thick, wrap it in plastic, and chill it in the refrigerator for at least 1 hour.

3 Turn out the dough onto a lightly floured surface. Using a floured rolling pin, roll the dough into a 10-inch (25 cm) round that is ¼ inch (6 mm) thick. Place the round on the prepared baking sheet.

4 To make the filling: Sprinkle the oat flour and salt over the pastry, leaving a 1-inch (2.5 cm) border uncovered at the edge. Spread the pecans in a 7-inch (18 cm) circle in the center of the dough. Arrange the apples in concentric circles over the nuts. Sprinkle the apples with the maple sugar. Bring the pastry up and over the apples to make a top crust, leaving the center uncovered. Dot the apples in the center with the butter.

5 Brush the top crust with the beaten egg mixture and sprinkle generously with the coarse sugar.

6 Bake the galette for 20 minutes, until golden brown. Remove from the oven and let it cool to lukewarm before serving.

WALDORF SALAD

YIELD: 6 SERVINGS

¼ cup (56 g) mayonnaise

¼ cup (38 g) Greek yogurt

3 tablespoons (45 ml) honey

1 tablespoon (15 ml) lemon juice

4 crisp green apples, peeled and diced

1½ cups (168 g) chopped walnuts

½ cup (76 g) grapes, halved, or raisins, depending on the season

Salt, to taste

Butter lettuce leaves

This is an old-fashioned dish, but it is the perfect snack. It is filled with healthy fats from the walnuts and nutrients from the fruits. The addition of Greek yogurt adds a little protein to the traditional recipe. Try to buy local honey, because it has been shown to help people reduce their allergy symptoms.

1   In a small mixing bowl, combine the mayonnaise, yogurt, honey, and lemon juice. Add salt to taste.

2   In a larger mixing bowl, combine the apples, walnuts, and grapes/raisins.

3   Pour the lemon dressing over the apple mixture and mix well. Salt to taste.

4   Serve atop lettuce leaves.

DATE AND WALNUT COOKIES

This is great project to make with children, because it's going to be messy no matter who makes it. It's very sweet, but as desserts go, it is healthy, because it is made with dates and walnuts. Dates have a lot of minerals and are high in fiber. The walnuts are filled with healthy Omega-3 fats, as well as minerals. The original recipe calls for white flour and a caramel glaze, but this version has less sugar and uses nutty almond flour, which adds its own sweetness.

YIELD: 30 COOKIES

30 pitted dates, sliced

1½ cups (168 g) large walnut halves

4 tablespoons (56 g) butter, softened

¾ cup (144 g) packed light brown sugar

1 egg, lightly beaten

½ cup (124 g) sour cream

1 cup (120 g) all-purpose flour

¼ cup (15 g) almond flour, finely ground

¼ teaspoon salt

¼ teaspoon baking powder

½ teaspoon baking soda

1   Preheat the oven to 400°F (200°C). Line 2 baking sheets with parchment paper.

2   Stuff each date half with a walnut piece and set aside.

3   In a small mixing bowl, beat the butter with the sugar until it is blended and smooth. Add the egg and mix well. Stir in the sour cream.

4   In a larger mixing bowl, combine the flours, salt, baking powder, and baking soda. Add the butter and sugar mixture to the flours and mix well.

5   Keeping a bowl of water nearby (to rinse your fingers), dip each stuffed date into the batter and place on cookie sheet. Leave space between cookies. Because of the shape, the batter won't be smooth around each date.

6   Bake for 8 to 10 minutes. Remove each cookie to a cooling rack after they have cooled for a minute or two. Store in an airtight container for up to three days. Do not refrigerate.

BANANA-APPLE BUCKWHEAT MUFFINS

YIELD: 12 MUFFINS

¾ cup (90 g) buckwheat flour

2 teaspoons (3 g) baking powder

½ teaspoon salt

3 large eggs

¼ cup (64 g) unsweetened applesauce

1 banana, mashed

⅓ cup (79 ml) honey

1½ cups (188 g) apple, peeled and diced

½ cup (56 g) walnuts, chopped

These are a great option for people who are gluten-free, because there is no white flour in this recipe. This recipe is also healthy because it contains no refined sugar. You can eat these for breakfast or take them along in a lunch box or on a hike. These keep well frozen, too. Just wrap them individually and then store.

1 Preheat the oven to 350°F (177°C) and line a muffin tin with paper liners.

2 Whisk together flour, baking powder, and salt. In another bowl, whisk together eggs, applesauce, banana, and honey.

3 Mix banana mixture into flour mixture, and then add apple and walnuts.

4 Pour batter into muffin cups. Bake about 30 minutes. Check with toothpick; it should come out clean when muffins are done.

5 Let cool to serve.

CONCLUSION

B eing "grounded" brings together the science of physics, biology, and psychology. It is not a New Age term, although it is a relatively young phrase. In fact, according to Merriam-Webster, the word *grounded* first appeared in 1958. Later, it became a metaphor for a feeling and a way of being. Wires were grounded before people were.

Fortunately, scientists now recognize the potential of grounding to improve health. In fact, in 2024, Arizona opened the first Grounding Park near Flagstaff.

Called The Barefoot Trail, its one mile (1.6 km) features a reflexology path, as well as information explaining why the locale is so beneficial. The park offers programs to help visitors best connect with the earth.

Of course, as you learned in this book, you can ground yourself wherever you are, even if you are far from nature.

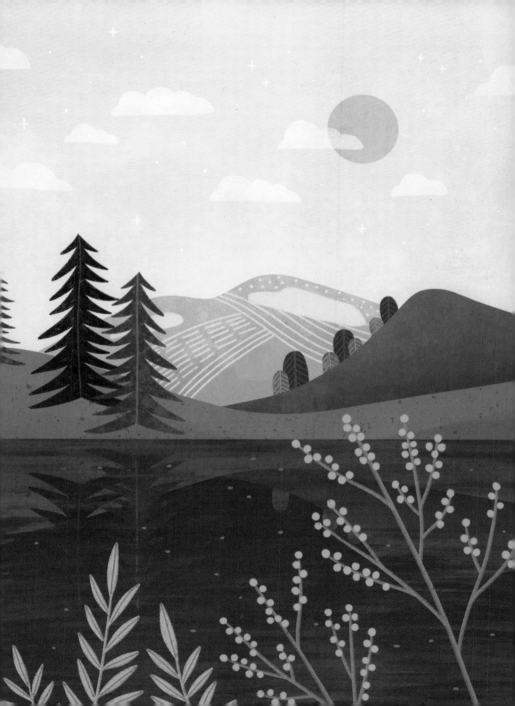

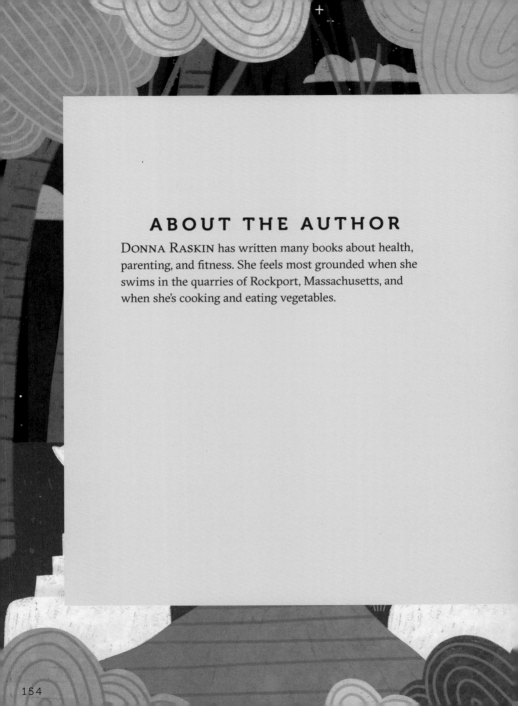

ABOUT THE AUTHOR

DONNA RASKIN has written many books about health, parenting, and fitness. She feels most grounded when she swims in the quarries of Rockport, Massachusetts, and when she's cooking and eating vegetables.

ACKNOWLEDGMENTS

Thank you to Jill Alexander, Winnie Prentiss, Anne Re, Meredith Quinn, Brooke Pelletier, Samantha Bednarek, Tiffany Hill, and Bea Müller for their vision and creativity.

INDEX